I0830344

LONGEVITY NOTES
2020

JACOB LINDAMAN

IOWA

JANUARY 2020

Longevity Notes 2020 by Jacob Lindaman

This book or the parts thereof my not be reproduced in any form stored in a retrieval system or transmitted in any form by any means – electronic, mechanical, photocopy, recording or otherwise – without prior written permission of the author except as provided by United States of America copyright law.

Cover art designed by Jacob Lindaman

First Edition
ISBN 978-1-79482-565-9

TABLE OF CONTENTS

FORWARD

This is a book about increasing longevity. Other books on this topic exist, but they usually falter in one of two ways; they are either too broad or too narrow in scope. Those that err in breadth do so by attempting to speak to every study, every supplement, every unvetted health claim leaving the reader with so much information that he can't do anything with it. The biggest problem with this type of mistake is that it often includes legitimate solutions, but they are indistinguishable from the piles of crap they are covered in. Usually, this sort of garbage is restricted to a blog, but on occasion it makes its way into print. When in print watch out for multiple titles reflecting popular health trends all by the same author.

The second err is when a book only sees one solution and ignores all other possibilities to increase longevity. The Blue Zones book is a fantastic report on a longevity study, but the author ignored several major contributing factors to increasing longevity. The result was an overemphasis of a plant-based diet. You might get hit by a bus or die from complications of a medication. A centuries old plant-based diet won't protect you from buses or doctor's prescriptive mistakes. Did you know the closer you live to an airport the more likely you are to have elevated levels of lead in your blood which is now known to lead to your demise? Plant-based diets are equally as useless at combating lead poisoning. Does your plant-based diet include food that was grown in a field sprayed with RoudUp (glyphosate)? RoundUp stays on the plants, gets inside of animals who eat it and ends up inside of you when you eat the plant or the animal that ate the plant. RoundUp has recently been shown to be the cause of liver disease.[1]

This book is different. If you wanted to live a long time wouldn't you want to know what you would eventually die from? You don't need a crystal ball. As it turns out most people die from just a few chronic illnesses. If you can prepare to avoid those chronic illnesses you will either delay their onset or avoid them completely so that when you finally die it will be from something else; probably an accident, but even fatal accidents can be minimized. When someone dies from an accident there are really just a few ways they die. Taking a moment to investigate this you can reduce your chances of this major cause of death as well.

Your health is your responsibility. You live in an age of unimaginable freedom and wealth. The house you live in is probably larger than the house your parents lived in at the same stage in life and they were the wealthiest generation the world had known until yours came along. Without a doubt you have electricity in your home, running water, trash pickup service, refrigeration, stove, oven, microwave, toaster, dishwasher, instant access to pretty much all the collective knowledge ever produced by humanity by using your phone or computer. Let's not forget your heating and air conditioning. I could go on, but I want you to realize that all these things you have are luxuries that no one else has ever dreamt about. Kings and queens of Europe, Emperors, Caesars and Pharaohs have never had what the middle-class Westerner has.

These luxuries are a gift from God. Not just to you, but you to them. God could have put you in the world 900 years ago or he could have put you into a world that doesn't have access to free libraries, free public education or texting. But He didn't. He gave you all of those things.

Have you ever wondered why God put you here; why He put you now? Those blessings mentioned above are for you to use. God invites you to participate in His grand scheme; you get to play. He's given you the gear. Do something with it. Use those luxuries to make the world better. You can live and learn and influence others with greater ease than anyone before you.

In the pages that follow you will read about longevity in a way you have never heard before. I encourage you to use this information to honor God by treating your body with respect. Your body is a gift from God. It is your honor to figure out how it works, maintain it, and put it to work for as long as possible.

Put it to work for as long as possible. The purpose of this book is to enable you to do that. The longer you live the more you can do.

LONGEVITY MATTERS

The best place to start is the beginning. In the book of Genesis, after God had finished creating the universe, He molded some dirt together to make the first human body, but it was just a body. In the next step God breathed His spirit into the body and voilà, it became a living soul.

The recipe the Bible gives us for human life is body + spirit = soul.

The body is confined to the physical world. The physical world is made of only 3 things; space, time and matter. The spirit is bound by the body until the body dies.

The purpose of the body is to house your personal spirit and the Holy Spirit and to interact with the physical world in a way the spirit cannot.

Longevity matters for 2 reasons;

1.)   Maintaining the body allows its user to worship God longer.

2.)   Taking care of the body is an act of responsible stewardship.

Both of the reasons mentioned above are acts of worship. For ages philosophers have pondered the meaning of man's existence. Millenia of searching and asking; working and hoping; scientific inquiry and fancy speech have all resulted in fruitless babble.

The meaning of life is to worship your Creator. Jesus Christ planned you, formed you, gave you your initial breath and asks that you worship Him as your Creator; as your Savior.

The choice is yours. Keep this in mind as you consider these words; a long life without Christ is no better than a short one with Him.

Over 2,700,000 people die each year in America. Almost 2,000,000 will die from one of the 9 illnesses discussed in this booklet. You are going to die someday. Just playing the odds you have about a 75% chance of dying from one of these 9 illnesses too. The vast majority of these deaths are from preventable illness caused by cerebrovascular accidents and diabetes.

Your health is important. It's also complicated, but it doesn't have to be. This book is organized into simple topics outlined with small doses of great information. Each chapter tackles 1 of the top 9 leading causes of death. You'll find uncommon ways to treat yourself and improve your health to avoid or at least prolong your life so you do not succumb to one of these 9 causes of death. Of the top 10 causes of death tracked by the CDC only suicide is not mentioned as it is a mental illness, but depression and anxiety will be addressed later. The scope of this little book is limited to physical illnesses.

Almost everything mentioned has been researched and studied; sources are listed. While I may mention a few products, it is for the purpose of education, to demonstrate a point or make you aware that you don't need to eat 50 pounds of blueberries every day to get enough pterostilbene. You can buy a supplement for $20 that will last you a month.

Grouping non-traditional approaches into an alternative therapy category tends to diminish the value of legitimate treatment options. Just because something isn't 'western medicine' does not mean its ineffective. I want to make it clear, however, that you won't be reading about essential oil cure-alls, homeopathic remedies or other over-hyped fad treatments; however, some of the treatments discussed could be considered alternative simply because they are not well known. This does not mean research invalidates their use. In fact, you will see, that many of them have been shown to be effective through scientific inquiry. Some of them are fairly new so they haven't had the time to become well known.

The CDC estimates that each year about 40% of deaths are from preventable causes. In other words, at least 40% of people who died didn't have to. They died from self-inflicted diseases. This estimate should probably be higher based on how diabetes is considered. I would say that most of the 1.9 million deaths from chronic illnesses are largely preventable. Historically, smoking has been responsible for the most preventable deaths. Soon, it will be obesity.

It didn't used to be like this. After World War II American life changed, for economic reasons beyond the scope of this book, in one grand way that underlies everything about our society today – we were wealthier. Europe's economy was destroyed. This led businesses and governments to invest in America. With the whole world investing in one place money seemed to grow on trees. Everyone had a good paying job. Everyone could afford their basic necessities and a few new luxury items. Many businesses developed amazing scientific discoveries originally used for war. Once it was over they were ready to sell these in new markets directed at the public instead of the government. This was the era of microwaves, tv dinners, televisions, suburban neighborhoods, office parks, cars for every family, interstate highways, commute times, office jobs instead of labor jobs, plastics replacing metals and lots and lots of cheap food.

Stop for a minute. Have you ever wondered what life was like before these changes? You may have pondered how people lived back then.

But have you ever considered how they died?

Even though recordkeeping was not then what it is now we can see that the causes of death are different. Today, the vast majority of deaths can be contributed to overeating and underutilizing the body. Because people back then were poorer they bought less food and the food they ate was diverse. (I would even argue that a medieval peasant had a healthier diet than the average American reading this. More on that later.) They were more physically active which meant they burned more calories and built more muscle. Physical activity does much more to benefit your health than simply build muscle. If these people weren't as overweight as us and they got a good deal of exercise what killed them?

The leading causes of death from the 1800's look nothing like they do today. The top ten killers were all infectious diseases. The older you got the more likely you were to die from an infection. Not from cancer. Not heart disease. Not strokes. Not diabetes. They were infections. While many people today die from infections and many people in the 1800's died from cancers and circulatory ailments the ratios today have flipped. When people aged they didn't wear down in the same way we wear down today.

Their lack of understanding germ theory exposed them to more germs and we've developed effective ways to treat infections. This means we now live in a world where deadly infections have largely been reduced. Everything from clean water in the home to implementing effective sewage removal has impacted how we treat cleanliness. Even children understand how germs work. We wash our hands. We sterilize surgical instruments. We use chemicals that kill germs. Vaccines have saved millions. Victory is ours.

But if we are truly victorious *why don't we live any longer?*

Let me expand on that; people today, living in a modern scientific society don't live any longer than any prior generation whose living conditions were on par with a third world country. People had the same life expectancy as us who lived in log cabins, had dirt floors, spent hours each day preparing meals, rode horses or walked to their destinations, dwelled in cities with no running water, no sewer system, didn't understand what a calorie was, didn't save for retirement or enroll their children in the finest schools. You can probably expand it to not just the early days of America, but all the way through the Medieval Period and beyond. The fact that we don't live longer than them is debatable, but there is evidence to support it. We moderns have dramatically reduced the infant mortality rate (mostly from understanding how germs spread and sanitizing equipment used for delivering babies) which in turn has increased life expectancy. However, and this is my point, if you were born in 1835 and survived being born you were likely to live until about 75 years old. Now, you can expect to live to about 77. Hats off to improving infant mortality, but for the rest of us that's not much improvement. In fact, you are less likely to make it to the century mark than someone living in 100 B.C.

Back to the big question; if we aren't dying from the same things why aren't we living longer?

Remember those dramatic lifestyle changes after World War II? They led to a life of ease. No need to worry about food. No need for physical labor. Food now comes from the fridge. Labor is for someone else or increasingly, for a machine. Let someone else mow your yard, fix your car, plow your driveway, make your food, clean your home. One of the biggest changes taking place is that grocery stores are implementing a way for you to order your groceries online. They will pick them out and deliver them to your door. Gone are the days of pushing a cart from aisle to aisle. Let someone else do that. And more so we are using machines to replace the physical labor that even hired hands once performed.

That's where we are today. That is the typical, average, expected; the status quo and this attitude leads to a typical and expected death. Are you surprised that people who live and act just like everyone else die from the same causes at the same age?

You don't have to be like everyone else. Look around you. Look at all the things that everyone does that makes them a copy. I'm not asking you to be a different person, but I am asking you to question what you see. Is this the way life is supposed to be?

I don't think so. I don't accept as truth the way the world presents itself to me. I don't want to kill myself with the ignorance of germ theory that our ancestors died from. I don't want to kill myself from the ignorance of self-inflicted diseases that my generation is dying from. This is not a book that yearns for the past and wishes things would be the way they used to be. Instead, let's look to the past and see the value that is there and meld that with new knowledge to improve our lives.

What follows is a list of the leading causes of death in America. This list started out as a way for me to identify novel treatments and preventative measures for these diseases that, for one reason or another, are effective, but not well known. I've mentioned that I'm not going to preach voodoo science or try to sell you something. You also won't hear the oft repeated eat a balanced diet, don't smoke, increase your antioxidants, reduce stress and many other nuggets of typically good, though incomplete advice on how to be healthy. A marketing slogan isn't going to save your life. What you will read about are ways, you have more than likely never heard of, to combat the diseases that are killing us. For example, you know what vitamin K is, but have you ever heard of vitamin K_2? It's different, lacking from our diet and research demonstrates that it is very very important. So is cholesterol and saturated fat. Did you know type II diabetes can be cured…easily? And what about the big mother of them all – cancer. No, I haven't found the cure, but there are novel ways to reduce your likeliness of developing cancer that are backed by simple evidence.

One last thing; almost everything discussed here is pretty cheap and can be done without a prescription, surgical procedure or any other expert's guidance – there are a few exceptions. Basically, you can do this stuff yourself and you can afford it. Having said that I will also caution you that if you are unsure, unhealthy, or feel that you don't fully understand what you're reading then you should probably first talk to a knowledgeable physician. They will be the ones to know if something is not right with you. The purpose of this book is to house my collection of thoughts organized into notes. *This book is for me*, but you are welcome to look through it. Use it as a starting point to get ideas that *you* research further. This is my disclaimer. Know your limits. Ask questions. Learn about your body. This book will not diagnose or treat you. It only offers some ideas to explore. Your health is your responsibility.

Want to get better? Start exploring.

LEADING CAUSES OF DEATH

1850	**2016**
1.) Tuberculosis	1.) Heart disease
2.) Dysentery/diarrhea	2.) Cancer
3.) Cholera	3.) Accidents
4.) Malaria	4.) Chronic Lower Resp Disease
5.) Typhoid Fever	5.) Stroke
6.) Pneumonia	6.) Alzheimer's Disease
7.) Diphtheria	7.) Diabetes
8.) Scarlet Fever	8.) Influenza
9.) Meningitis	9.) Kidney Disease
10.) Whooping Cough	10.) Suicide

HEART DISEASE 635,260 & STROKE 142,142 COMBINED 777,402

The medical world treats heart disease by emphasizing a reduction in cholesterol from the diet and blood serum, reducing fat, especially saturated fat, and sodium from the diet as well. These efforts are inadequate to properly treat heart disease as a whole and ignore the entirety of a person's health. Every single one of these is a nutrient your body needs. By eliminating or suppressing them expect to see repercussions elsewhere in your body.

The main issue with heart disease is plaque formation in the arteries; it restricts blood flow and increases blood pressure. This usually results in narrowing the lumen - inside of the artery - which restricts blood flow.

Plaques form through progressive stages. The earliest stage involve some sort of lesion to the endothelial lining on the inside of the artery. Official cardiologist theories are not 100% certain what causes this lesion; continuing with their theory is that cholesterol is somehow involved. Eventually, high serum cholesterol causes a heart attack despite the fact that cholesterol is only a minor player in plaque composition. A plaque can continue to grow until it is capped off with a layer of calcium. At this point the clot has been growing for decades and begins to present serious symptoms.

This is a simplification of traditional thinking on how an artery clogs. It is only to provide insight. The main points to remember are that A.) this is caused over a long period of time, B.) calcium is involved in the later stages and C.) the mantra falsely blames cholesterol when we should be looking elsewhere.

I've combined heart disease with strokes as the vast majority of each of these has virtually the same pathology. The resulting symptom manifests itself in different locations; a clot forms in a cardiac artery or an artery in the brain. Clots can even form in other locations such as organs. Wherever they form the disease progression results in a clot obstructing blood flow.

In the real world there are 4 steps to cardiovascular disease.

> 1.) Endothelial damage
> 2.) Clot formation or dysfunctional clot formation
> 3.) Clot repair or dysfunctional clot repair
> 4.) The final clot

Anything that addresses any of these steps will improve outcomes. I've organized the following section to show strategies that work, but maybe haven't been demonstrated to have a specific benefit. This is followed by a section with strategies addressing each of the 3 steps (you can't do anything about the 4th step; death). The lists are not all inclusive; there could be thousands of entries. A great deal of this information is taken from the blog of Dr. Malcolm Kendrick.[2]

The innermost layer of the endothelium is called the glycocalyx. It is composed of many hairs which serve to lubricate the surface keeping blood flowing freely and protect the cells beneath. The endothelium manufactures nitric oxide which helps to dilate blood vessels. Damage to the endothelium will reduce nitric oxide production which in turn will reduce the ability of the blood vessel to dilate when it should.

ENDOTHELIAL DAMAGE
A list of things that damage endothelium or prevent its formation

Air Pollution
Albumin low levels
Angiotensin II
Blood Pressure high levels
Diabetes/High Blood Sugar
Dehydration
Erythema Nodosum
Infection/Sepsis
Kidney Disease
Lead – chelation therapy to remove lead.
Mercury – chelation therapy to remove mercury.
Migraine
Oral Steroids
Proton Pump Inhibitors

Renin Aldosterone Angiotensin System activation
Rheumatoid Arthritis
Scleroderma
Smoking
Stress Hormones
Vitamin B Deficiency
Vitamin C Deficiency

NITRIC OXIDE
A list of substances that increase NO

Albumin
Exercise
l-arginine
l-citrulline
Lycopene
Meditation
Potassium
Sunshine
Vitamin C
Vitamin D

CLOT FORMATION
A list of things that increase clot formation

Dehydration
Diabetes/High Blood Sugar
Fibrinogen high levels
       Alcohol reduces fibrinogen levels.
Lipoprotein (a) high levels
NSAIDs
Plasminogen Activator Inhibitor 1 high levels
Stress hormones
VLDL/triglycerides high levels

       Aspirin reduces clotting.
       HDL Cholesterol reduces clotting.
       Omega 3's reduce clotting.

CLOT REPAIR
A list of things that impair clot repair

Plasminogen activator inhibitor 1 (PAI-1) high levels
Plasminogen tissue activator (TPa) breaks apart clots.

The following is a list of remedies for circulatory disease. These may benefit either heart disease, stroke or both. This list is not all inclusive and is intended as an attempt to prevent disease and promote health for these systems.

1.)   VITAMIN K_2 – Removes calcium plaques from arteries & deposits them in bone.[3] K_2 is present in Natto & supplements. There are different forms of Vitamin K_2. Menaquinone appears to be the most effective.

2.)   DON'T SMOKE.

3.)   GARLIC – Preferably raw garlic. 2 cloves per day per WH Foods. Garlic oils, supplements and other preparations do not convey the same benefits. Despite the name elephant garlic is not garlic.

4.)   CALORIC RESTRICTION - Reduce calorie consumption and have a healthy weight.

5.)   EXTENDED SITTING - Avoid sitting for long periods. This will help vascular return. Compression socks help. Exercise is not enough. When sitting you must stand up and move every so often.

6.)   HYDROLYZED COLLAGEN – When eaten strengthens blood vessels. It also lowers blood pressure.[4] Collagen is a protein. Proteins are large molecules the body must digest into small amino acids so that they are small enough to absorb. Proteins that are broken down all the way into individual amino acids, but still retain several amino acids bonded together, are called peptides. These are the same as collage that is hydrolyzed or partially digested. It has always been thought the body cannot absorb large molecules.

However, one creative study[5] provided radioactive collagen peptides to rats then measured if they absorbed any. Turns out they did. The study confirms that hydrolyzed collagen can be absorbed and provide health benefits.

7.)   EXERCISE – Get your heart rate up.

8.)   RESVERATROL – Rat studies show it improves vascular health, reduces LDL cholesterol oxidation, and protects the heart in a heart attack.[6] Hyperglycemia, as in diabetes, causes endothelial damage. Resveratrol prevents or reduces this damage.[7] 10mg of resveratrol per day for 3 months improved left ventricle function, endothelial function, lowered LDL cholesterol and protected hemorheological changes in patients with coronary artery disease.[8]

9.)   CALCIUM – Reduce calcium consumption from supplements. Increasing calcium does not prevent bone fractures in elderly. Once you reach the minimum amount your bones can use the rest of the calcium goes somewhere else in your body. This means it will increase the amount of calcium in your blood which contributes to plaque formation. This clogs arteries and contributes to heart attacks.[9] The same study also noted that those who had the highest amounts of calcium which came from their diets were least likely to have a heart attack while those who used supplements were most likely to have a heart attack. They believe this may reflect the participants' diets in general. Those who had the highest total calcium from their diet had a healthier diet. Those who only used the supplement had a poor diet.

Another study concluded, "*Calcium supplements with or without vitamin D marginally reduce total fractures but do not prevent hip fractures in community-dwelling individuals. They also cause kidney stones, acute gastrointestinal events, and increase the risk of myocardial infarction and stroke. Any benefit of calcium supplements on preventing fracture is outweighed by increased cardiovascular events. While there is little evidence to suggest that dietary calcium intake is associated with cardiovascular risk, there is also little evidence that it is associated with fracture risk.*" This further emphasizes that dietary calcium does not play a role in heart attacks or prevent broken bones, but supplements with calcium and even calcium and vitamin D increase the risk of heart attacks and do nothing to prevent broken bones.[10]

10.)   REDUCE INFLAMMATION – Several studies demonstrate measuring and then reducing levels of inflammation as an adequate treatment for heart disease. Inflammation is a sign that damage has occurred, but that healing is taking place. Simply reducing inflammation may not be the most effective measure. Rather, an attempt should be made to identify what is causing the damage and to prevent this. The body should be allowed to heal.

11.)   VITAMIN D_3 – Helps create nitric oxide which improves blood flow and removes clots. D_3 also reduces the level of oxidative stress on the cardiovascular system. Treatment with D_3 can restore endothelium in blood vessels back to normal. D_3 can help prevent heart attacks and treat those who have had them.[11]

12.)   LEAD EXPOSURE – Lead reduces the epithelial lining of blood vessels and causes hypertension by damaging kidneys. This increases the likelihood of plaque formation. Low levels of lead in the blood were once thought safe as symptoms arose in other areas; cognition, growth, etc. But now these lower levels have been found to contribute to deaths related to heart disease. Airplanes still use leaded gasoline. Those who live closer to airports have higher amounts of lead in their blood. Previously, estimated deaths from lead exposure were about 40,000 per year. However, after a recent study this figure is now estimated to be approximately 10x more than this. Lead exposure should probably be listed as one of the top 10 causes of death.[12]

13.)   SAUNA – 45 minutes/week in a sauna significantly reduces cardiovascular disease.[13] This is because your cells produce heat shock proteins in response to stress; heat, cold, UV light exposure and wound healing. Heat shock proteins help new proteins fold correctly which prevents disease.

14.) VO_2 MAX – People with a low VO_2 max are much more likely to develop cardiovascular disease and die than people with a greater VO_2 max. The only way to increase your VO_2 max is regular cardio. VO_2 max measures the maximum volume of oxygen used during exercise.

15.)   WALNUTS – Consumption of walnuts has long term positive effects for almost all areas of cardiovascular health.[14]

16.)   FRUCTOSE – Cut out fructose. Saturated fat is often cited as the culprit for high cholesterol. However, saturated fat is a diverse class of chemicals. Some have positive impacts on cholesterol levels. When saturated fat is replaced with sugar, specifically fructose, high-fructose corn syrup, sweeteners such as sucrose, etc. the result is a worse cholesterol profile.[15]

17.)   CALCIUM – While decreasing calcium consumption benefits heart disease it does not appear to impact the occurrence of strokes. Increasing milk intake correlates to a decrease in strokes. Calcium intake from nondairy sources is unrelated to stroke occurrence.[16]

18.)   DEHYDRATION – Dehydration damages endothelium and thickens blood encouraging it to clot. You are the most dehydrated in the morning as your kidneys have been filtering water out of your blood during the night and you have not consumed any liquids. Heart attacks are most common in the morning. This is frequently associated with high cortisol levels. Cortisol levels fluctuate naturally throughout the day following the circadian rhythm. They are highest in the morning. Cortisol causes blood vessels to vasoconstrict. The link between high morning cortisol and heart attacks is likely to be true, but and in additional to this, dehydration is also a major factor. Dehydration can also occur after periods of intense physical activity and neglect of replenishing fluids absent physical exertion.

> Drink a glass of water if you wake up in the night.
> Consume fluids first thing in the morning.
> Ensure you are well hydrated throughout the day.

One study showed that skipping breakfast lead to a significant increase in death. The authors stated they adjusted for many factors, but this is very difficult. Two things they did not account for were poverty and beverage consumption. It could be that poor people tend to eat less breakfast. Breakfast consumption then was measured as a proxy for poverty. The same can be said about beverage consumption. They may have measured that if people don't consume breakfast they tend to also not drink anything in the morning furthering their nocturnal state of dehydration.[17]

19.)   LYCOPENE + FAT + TOMATO – Has many benefits to cardiovascular and endothelial health. In the near future it will likely be considered an essential nutrient as it has repeatedly been shown that those who have low lycopene levels are significantly unhealthier than those with higher levels. 8g a day for as little as a few days to a few weeks markedly improves health. Lycopene is fat soluble and must be ingested alongside fat otherwise the body cannot absorb it.

20.)   RESTING HEART RATE – If your resting heart rate is over 75 beats per minute and you are 50 years old you are twice as likely to die from a heart attack than if your heart rate was 55 beats per minute.[18]

21.)   SODIUM – All humans in all cultures gravitate towards about 3-4 grams of sodium per day. This is about 8-10 grams of salt. Reducing salt consumption increases your resting heart rate which means your heart must work harder. Over time this extra effort can cause the heart to grow larger and become less flexible making each pump less efficient. This, in turn, forces the heart to pump even harder. And so goes the circle until after years and years of compounding problems it gives out. Most of this info was taken from the book The Salt Fix.

Many studies examining sodium intake conclude that high salt diets are unhealthy. Approach these carefully. There is much to be said about what is being measured and what is being reported. There is no standard definition for low salt intake, high salt intake, etc. So, this can vary from one study to the next. Also, assessing the health of those who consume large amounts of salt can direct researchers to misleading conclusions. Salt almost always accompanies calories. While it may be true that those who consume a lot of salt may be unhealthy it might actually be an excess of calories that causes the disease rather than the salt.

22.)   SILICON – Silicon is a little-known nutrient. Your body doesn't need much of it, but it is very important. It is found in high concentrations in connective tissue such as bone, skin, trachea and the aorta. The lowest levels are in the liver, heart, muscle and lung. "*It is therefore plausible to assume that observed decrease of silicon concentration in the aging population may be linked to several disorders, including atherosclerosis.*"[19]

CANCER 598,038

GENERAL CANCER STRATEGIES

Cancer is the number 2 killer in America. This alone makes it of great concern to everyone. You maybe have a family member who died from cancer. You won't get to far in this world without knowing someone who has died from it. Cancer seems to be everywhere.

Let's take a step back and look at some numbers. Of the almost 600,000 cancer deaths the largest is from lung cancer with about 150,000. The CDC estimates that 80-90% of these are caused by smoking. Radon exposure is responsible for almost all of the rest. Don't smoke and put in a modest effort to mitigate radon (or live in an area of the country where this is not a concern) and lung cancer is no longer of any worry.

After lung cancer is colorectal cancer with 52,000 deaths. Colorectal cancer is one of the easiest cancers to detect and treat.

The next biggest cancer killers are breast and prostate at about 41,000 each. While this is a large number it is not large enough to rank in the top 10. In fact, if we remove smoking the only cancer in the top 10 is colorectal cancer and it just barely edges out kidney disease.

Avoiding cancer is important, but it is easy to be overwhelmed without a proper perspective. My hope is that you will make efforts to avoid cancer, but also not fester on the larger 600,000 number. 6000,000 Americans do not die every year from one particular cancer.

The following strategies address multiple forms of cancer or have been shown to reduce cancer incidence in general rather than targeting a specific form of cancer.

1.)   REDUCE SUGAR - Reduce sugar consumption to starve 50% of cancers (how does this effect skin cancers?). The body breaks down most carbohydrates into glucose. Most cancer cells obtain ATP (energy) through glycolysis, splitting glucose into pyruvate and H+ with or without the presence of oxygen. This is called the Warburg Effect. Reducing ingestion of carbohydrates which your body converts to glucose limits the main source of energy for cancer cells thus starving them to death.

2.)   DON'T SMOKE

3.)   RESVERATROL – Can prevent cancer by fixing DNA that was not copied properly.

4.)   PTEROSTILBENE - Is even more potent than resveratrol.

5.)   CALORIC RESTRICTION – Reducing the amount of food you eat reduces the amount of reactive oxygen species you create. Think of this as simply losing weight. Count your calories and weigh yourself every day. If you gained weight eat fewer calories. If you lost weight then eat about the same number of calories. If you are really active you will burn more calories.
      Avoid metabolic rate calculators as there exists great variation on people's basal metabolic rate. The calculators maybe ok to get a rough idea of what could be going on, but don't rely on them.

6.)   EXERCISE – Increases energy demands on your body which forces mitochondria to create more energy. As a byproduct of this energy they create reactive oxygen species which causes cells to die. This is a normal process which prevents older damaged cells from multiplying and turning cancerous.

7.)   SLEEP – Sleep increases the production of cancer killer T cells. Poor sleep reduces the number of killer cells. Sleep disruption could be considered carcinogenic.

8.)   HYPERTHERMIA TREATMENTS – Raising body temp to 103. Can be done on localized tissue with higher temps. Cells develop resistance to heat. They take 3 – 4 days to lose this resistance. Treatment should be done no more than 2 times per week. Heating lasts about an hour. Should be done with a physician's guidance.

9.)   ALLERGIES – Allergy sufferers have 50% less incidence of cancer than non-allergy sufferers. This is thought to be because IgE antibodies cling to pollen, dust, etc., but don't seem to function outside of this. The current theory is that IgE antibodies also cling to cancer cells. Allergy sufferers produce more IgE antibodies than nonallegery sufferers. Avoid allergy medication if you can as these reduce IgE antibodies.

10.)   REDUCE IRON – Iron is food for tumors. Over time elevated iron levels are a significant factor in cancer incidence. Even iron levels at the middle and high end of what is typically considered safe can contribute to tumorigenesis. Test your ferritin levels to know what your iron is. Hemoglobin is not the same as ferritin.

Most labs consider a normal ferritin range to be 20-500ng/ml for men and 20-300ng/ml for women. A healthy range is probably more like 20-80ng/ml. Having ferritin levels at 490 doesn't give you any more energy or make you any healthier than someone who has a level of 40. Why expose yourself unnecessarily to something that could cause harm in the long term?

Iron is also a major oxidizing agent. It can alter DNA and damage healthy tissue.

There are only a few things you can do to reduce ferritin levels. The best thing is blood donation. This can reduce ferritin by about 20ng/ml with each donation. Avoid consuming iron rich foods. When consuming iron you can also consume other foods that prevent iron absorption such as coffee, tea, milk, phytates, etc.

11.)   WALNUTS – Have been shown to reduce breast, prostate and colorectal cancers. There are several biochemicals in walnuts that most likely work synergistically to slow tumor growth or reduce it. This is from mouse models which include mouse tumors and human tumors grafted onto mice.[20] 2 ounces a day is enough to slow breast cancer growth in mice.[21]

12.)   COFFEE – Dark roasted coffee decreased DNA breaks a lot.[22] Another study confirmed the same thing about coffee.[23]

13.)   BONE BROTH – Bone broth rich in cartilage contains antiangiogenesis factors that prevent formation of the small blood vessels tumors create to feed themselves. It also increases immune system function by causing it to produce more natural killer cells, T cells, B cells, B lymphocytes and antibodies. Even more, cartilage rich bone broth contains glycosaminoglycans that adhere to the cell membrane of tumors preventing them from replicating.

14.)   POMIFERIN – It is cytotoxic to many cancer cell lines; kidney, lung, prostate, breast, melanoma and colon which were tested. *"Histone deacetylase (HDAC) inhibitors have been identified that inhibit proliferation and induce differentiation and/or apoptosis of tumor cells in culture and in animal models."*[24]

The study reports the effectiveness of pomiferin and osajin to inhibit cancer cell growth, but measures them individually and concludes that a synthetic drug, suberoylanilide hydroxyamic acid (SAHA) was more effective. However, pomiferin and osajin occur together in the fruit of the Osage Orage (*Maclura pomifera*). Do these two substances possess synergistic properties?

15.)   CURCUMIN – In small amounts curcumin prevents DNA mutations and forces cancer cells into apoptosis; a natural process of programmed cell death that they normally suppress.

16.)   APPLE PEELS – Contain a substance that reactivates a tumor suppression gene that cancer cells have turned off.

SPECIFIC CANCER STRATEGIES

The following strategies are categorized according to specific cancer types. Occasionally, some strategies may overlap into two or more different cancer treatments, but because I haven't found anything to show them to be specific to a wider variety of cancers I've listed them here. Figures used for deaths come from the CDC.[25]

Cancer rates for Iowa closely match the national trends. There isn't anything specific to Iowa that deserves any special attention as far as prevention goes. The only possible exception would be radon exposure causing lung cancer. Other states may have higher rates of smoking which are the cause of their lung cancers. Iowans may suffer from lung cancer, at similar rates to the rest of the country, because of radon exposure. About 6,500 Iowans die each year from cancer.

LUNG CANCERS – 153,000   26%

The lungs interact with oxygen perhaps more than any other bodily tissue. Oxygen is highly corrosive making it an oxidizing agent. This is what antioxidants work to neutralize. Not all antioxidants are created equally. The lungs seem to prefer lycopene which happens to be one of the most powerful antioxidants.

Smoking alters the air entering the lungs increasing the oxidizing potential. Smoking is by far the largest contributor to lung cancer deaths. The CDC estimates that 80-90% of lung cancer deaths are caused by smoking. That would leave about 15,000 – 30,000 deaths from other causes and make lung cancer of minor concern as the 10th leading cause of cancer death.

1.)   RADON – After smoking radon is responsible for perhaps more lung cancer deaths than any other cause; about 20,000 annually. It is a radioactive material present mostly in Northern homes. It is colorless and odorless. You can hire a professional to measure the levels in your home or buy a DIY kit. If you have high levels there are several options you can pursue. The same crew who tested your home will probably also install radon mitigation systems. Typically, this involves a pump that pulls air from below your basement slab and moves it out of the house. They can also seal any cracks in the basement or crawlspace to ensure the pump works efficiently. Other strategies include opening the windows when the weather is conducive for this and liberal usage of ceiling fans. Ceiling fans push radon down where it can stick to dust and not be inhaled. Granite countertops give off a small amount of radon. Phosphate lawn fertilizers also contain radon. Radon is mostly a problem in the Midwest.

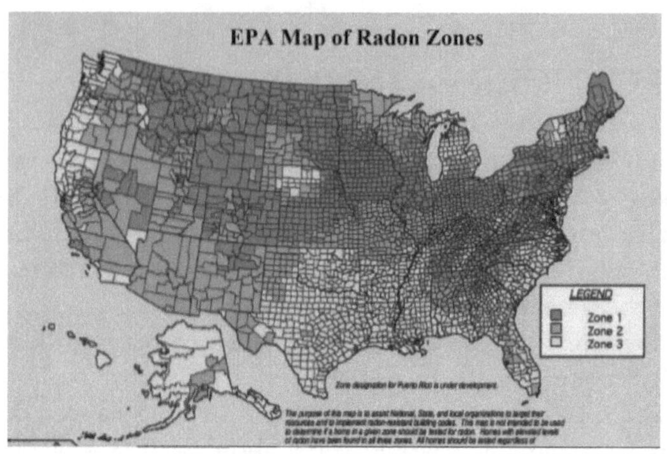

2.)   LYCOPENE – Lung tissue accumulates lycopene more than other antioxidants. β-carotene is another antioxidant found in the lungs. Both work well to protect the lungs from cancer. Smoking seems to transform these antioxidants into harmful substances which contribute to lung cancer formation.[26] Smoking could cause high levels of iron in the lungs which oxidize and cause disease.

3.)   SMOKING – Smoking is responsible for 80% - 90% of lung cancer deaths which is about 135,000 people per year. There is evidence that those with high ferritin/iron levels are much more likely to develop lung cancer if they smoke. Another way to think of this is if you smoke you are more likely to develop lung cancer if you also have high iron levels. Smoking may make iron more reactive so that it causes lung cancer.

COLORECTAL CANCER - 52,000   9%

Get checked. Colorectal cancer is one of the easiest forms of cancer to diagnose and treat.

1.)   EXTENDED SITTINGS - Avoid extended sitting. Sitting for just 2 hours at a time significantly increases cancers of the colon and rectum.[27] One of the shortfalls acknowledged by the authors is that people tend to eat more when sitting which could lead to adverse health outcomes. The conclusion then could be that those who eat more get colorectal cancers and those who sit for extended periods and do not eat more are just fine.

2.)   FIBER – If you read about fiber you will eventually come across some studies showing that ancient man or paleo man ate something like 50 or 100 grams of fiber per day. The conclusion is always that we should strive for this too. While the average American would benefit from increasing fiber consumption there is no reason to believe that such large amounts produced optimal health in any human. These studies on ancient people are usually based on a few teeth or incomplete skeletons found around a midden. All the dietary and health status conclusions are speculative at best. Should we strive to live like people who had a supposed life expectancy in the upper twenties?

Having said this, fiber does show a benefit to colon health. Shoot for 20 - 30 grams/day.

BREAST CANCER female - 41,500   7%

About half of the deaths from heart disease and stroke are females which is about 350,000 deaths per year. Note that breast cancer kills only about 10% of this figure. While breast cancer is a serious issue a woman should be far more concerned with heart cardiovascular health.

1.)   CHLORINE AVOIDANCE – Chlorine has been found in large amounts in breast tissue in women who have breast cancer. It isn't present in women who don't have breast cancer. Chlorine filters for showers and baths remove this. Avoid swimming pools and hot tubs. A chlorine filter for the shower costs about $30 and can be installed with very little handyman knowledge. Another filter for the bathtub or sink is the same price and even easier to install. Both can be purchased on Amazon. If you showered every day the filters would last about a year. You absorb more chemicals in a 10-minute shower than by drinking a gallon of water.

2.)   BIRTH CONTROL – There is an elevated risk for women to get breast cancer if they have taken birth control pills especially if they contain the drug progestin. 68 women out of 100,000 who took birth control will get breast cancer compared to 55 women out of 100,000 for the general population. An increase of 13 is about a 25% change. (13/55=23.6%). 10 million American women take birth control. This means 1,300 women will likely get breast cancer that otherwise would not have. Women who were on birth control pills for 10 years or more had an even higher risk of getting breast cancer.[28]

3.)   WALNUTS – 2 ounces of walnuts a day has amazing breast benefits.[29]

PANCREATIC CANCER – 41,000   7%

1.)   PANCREATIC CANCER MICROBIOME – All pancreatic cancer patients have the same microbiome which is significantly different than other people. Could this reflect a dietary cause rather than a microbiome source?

2.)   CURCUMIN – Large doses can treat pancreatic cancer.

3.)   FBL-03G – A non-psychoactive component of marijuana has shown promise to treat pancreatic cancer.[30]

PROSTATE CANCER – 29,000 5%

LIVER & BILE DUCT CANCER – 26,000   4%

This has doubled from 1999 – 2015.

LEUKEMIAS – 23,000   4%

1.)   BONE BROTH – I would love to see a study done on bone broth rich in bone marrow for leukemia patients. The only evidence that it is beneficial is anecdotal reports. Worst case scenario, if you have leukemia it wouldn't hurt to eat bone marrow.

NON-HODGKINS LYMPHOMA – 20,000 3%

BRAIN & NERVOUS SYSTEM – 16,200   3%

1.)   POMEFERIN – Extracted from the Osage Orange fruit, pomeferin has been shown to stop the growth of gliomas.[31]

BLADDER CANCER – 16,000   3%

1.)   COXSACKIEVIRUS – This virus is responsible for the common cold. It is inserted into the bladder with a catheter. It triggers an immune response that targets bladder cancer cells.[32] Is the immune system ineffective at reaching the bladder?

ESOPHAGEAL CANCER – 15,000   3%

1.)   HOT DRINKS – Hot drinks are strongly associated with cancers of the mouth and throat. While this truth has been accepted for some time the actual temperature of the drink has not been established. One study acknowledged this and sought to work out a rough figure. Their discovery was that tea hotter than 140°F doubled the occurrence of esophageal cancer in those who do not smoke or drink alcohol (confounding factors in other studies).[33]

2.)   STRAWBERRIES – 2 ounces of freeze-dried strawberries or 1 pound of fresh strawberries reversed precancerous esophageal cancer in 80% of patients. Half were disease free after 6 months.

KIDNEY & PELVIS – 14,500   2%

1.)   OCHRATOXIN A – See TESTICULAR CANCER.

OVARY CANCER – 14,000   2%

MYELOMA – 14,000   2%

STOMACH CANCERS – 11,000   2%

1.)   GARLIC – Prevents cancer of upper GI tract. Raw garlic is a better choice than cooked or garlic spices. Elephant garlic is not garlic.

2.)   SODIUM – Studies show that diets high in salt are likely to develop stomach cancer. However, the term 'high salt' is not universally defined. What you may think of as a lot of salt the researchers may not. Also, eating a lot of salt could be used as a proxy for eating a lot of food. Could an increase in calories be the true cause of these stomach cancers? One thing is for sure, if you hear about the evils of salt in a news story about a recent study be sure to look further into that study yourself. Average intake should be around 3 – 4 grams/day.

UTERUS & CORPUS, NOS – 10,000   2%

MELANOMA CANCERS – 9,000   2%

1.)   SAFE SUNSCREEN - Safe sunscreens that use zinc oxide or titanium dioxide. Ingredients other than this are extremely harmful. Most have been banned from tropical islands as they destroy reef habitats.

Brace yourself. Here comes a plug for essential oils…carrot seed oil has an spf of 40. Whew, no it doesn't cure skin cancer, but it is perfectly natural, cheap and chalk full of vitamin A. Please note, you don't smell it like most essential oil 'practitioners' advise for their oils. Pure carrot seed oil is pretty harsh stuff. You dilute it with another oil to make it a little gentler for your skin and then rub it on the area just like sunscreen. Other essential oils have good SPF values too, but carrot seed oil is by far the best. Surf shirts are lighter fabric with a special weave that gives them an spf of 50. This is a good option for people who are going to be outside sweating and want to stay cool. Cover up with hats, and long sleeve shirts.

2.)   INCREASE SKIN SPF - Eat foods to increase spf of skin. Dark skin is about 13 spf. Light skin is about 6 spf. Dark skin takes 13 times longer to burn than light skin. So, even a small increase in skin spf will go a long way.

   A.) *RETINOIDS* – *Lutein/Zeaxanthin* – Significantly prevents the formation of reactive oxygen species. Astaxanthin speeds up healing from Sun damage.

   Lycopene - 5 tablespoons of tomato paste over 3 months increases sunburn protection 40% or spf of about 3. Also, 40g of tomato paste which was calculated to include about 16mg of lycopene over 10 weeks reduced sunburn 40%. Must be taken with oil to increase absorption.[34] Also, lycopene by itself doesn't do much. It must be consumed with oil to be absorbed and also tomato products as there are other as yet to be identified substances in tomatoes that act synergistically with lycopene.

Beta carotene - 10 weeks added spf 4 to skin. Taken longer will add more spf. Unknown mechanism of action. Takes 1 – 2 months to develop hypercarotenemia at 20mg/day of beta carotene. A carrot has 4 mg.

Vitamin E 14 mg

Omega 3

Polypodium leucotomos – Multiple studies have shown oral ingestion of *polypodium leucotomos* increases the skin's ability to avoid damage from ultraviolet light. *Polypodium leucotomos* is a fern native to the eastern shores of South American, the Caribbean and Georgia and Florida in North America. It does not tolerate frost or temperatures just above freezing. The plant has been reclassified after initial studies demonstrated its many health benefits. It is now properly called *Phlebodium aureum*; however, the supplement industry grew out of the initial classification of *Polypodium leucotomos* and has not changed. It is generally considered safe. Take anywhere from 480mg/day to 1,200mg/day for several weeks.[35, 36]

B.) BEC/Solasodine rhamnosyl glycosides – For non-melanoma skin cancers. This is one of the more interesting treatments I've ever found because it appears to actually remove, ahem… 'cure' cancer. An extract from the Solanaceae family; eggplant, tomato, potato, bell peppers, tobacco. BEC5 is comprised of 1/3 solasonine, 1/3 solamargine and 1/3 rhamnose. Rhamnose is a sugar that attaches to the 2 extracts. The sugar binds to a receptor on a cancerous cell. The cancerous cell sees the sugar and lets the whole molecule in (see the glycolysis explanation above). This allows the other 2 components to get inside the cell and kill it. Without a sugar molecule attached to the extracts they cannot get inside the cell. Cancer cells live mostly from glycolysis which means they love sugar and have many sugar receptors. Make your own or order from a company called Curaderm. I've been watching this treatment for a few years. It started off as an amateur presentation that promised great results. But over time it seems to have gained more momentum from legitimate medical professionals. The amateurism, I assume, had to do with the fact that the developer of the BEC5 cream was more of a scientist than a marketing guru or businessman. As the cream proven itself the website, endorsements and more importantly the research are all validating its effectiveness. I've made my own concoction by peeling skins from eggplants and soaking in vinegar. Soak gauze in this mixture and apply it to your skin a few times a day.

C.) Antioxidants – Several studies show many skin diseases are associated with reduced antioxidant production. Application of antioxidants to the skin can drastically reduce tumor incidence. Antioxidant enzymes present on the skin include; glutathione reductase, catalase and superoxide dismutase. Manganese superoxide dismutase is often significantly reduced in hyperproliferative keratinocyetes in squamous cell carcinoma, basal cell epithelioma and benign hyperproliferative keratinocytes in psoriatic epidermis[37,38].

D.) Topical Retinoids – Retinoids such as vitamin A applied topically prevent damage from UV rays and also help to repair damage (this might explain how carrot seed oil works). Restores collagen formation and thickens collagen in photodamaged skin. Takes 4 to 6 months with tretinoin medication at 0.05% concentration. 0.01% concentration was much less effective, but still noticeable.[39, 40]

3.)   UV SCREENS – An ultraviolet light screen can easily be installed on windows. You can cut them to the size you need and stick them on. Be mindful when installing them. You need UV light to live. Placing UV filters everywhere could deprive you of the benefits you can only get from light. They would probably work best in locations where you are constantly exposed to sunlight and have no other options; if you drive a vehicle or sit in direct sunlight in an office building.

CERVICAL CANCER – 4,200   <1%

LARYNX CANCER – 3,700   <1%

MESOTHELIOMA – 2,500   <1%

1.)   ASBESTOS – Seems to be the only cause of mesothelioma.

THYROID CANCER – 1,900   <1%

1.)   RADIATION – Exposure to ionizing radiation, especially at a young age, has a strong correlation to thyroid cancer.

2.)   NITRATES – Consumption of nitrates from drinking water has a strong correlation to thyroid cancer. Nitrates compete with iodine for absorption. About 100% of men and women who died at 70 years of age had microscope tumors in their thyroids. That 100% figure could be less in people who are healthy enough to live longer than 70 years.

HODGKIN LYMPHOMA – 1,100   <1%

1.)   AVOID EPSTEIN-BARR INFECTION – 50% of Hodgkin Lymphomas are caused by the Epstein-Barr virus. 50% of 5-year-olds and 90% of adults have had an Epstein-Barr infection. It remains in the body for life. Epstein-Barr virus is the same virus that causes mononucleosis. It is estimated that 200,000 cancer cases a year are caused by Epstein-Barr. It is spread primarily by saliva.

2.)   BONE BROTH – Improves immune system function by increasing natural killer cells, T cells, B cells and antibodies. All of these help with Epstein-Barr/mono infection.

TESTICULAR CANCER – 400   <1%

1.)   OCHRATOXIN A – A carcinogenic mycotoxin produced by several molds; Aspergillus ochraceus, Aspergillus niger and Aspergillus carbonarius, Penicillium verrucosum, and species of Penicillium, Petromyces, and Neopetromyces. Human exposure to these microbes occurs in homes or buildings with water damage. The mycotoxin is airborne and easily inhaled. It can collect on air filters, water filters, duct work, Also, they tend to grow on several popular foods; coffee beans, grains, non-ruminant animals that eat grains – mostly pigs. While not present in beef as cows are ruminants whose digestive tract can breakdown ochratoxin A it is present in cow's milk.[41]

Ochratoxin A has mostly been studied in kidney disease, but has been shown to cause testicular cancer.[42] It is present in many tissues. One study hypothesized its occurrence in young males to correspond to testicular cancer. Phenylalanine and aspartame may protect against its toxicity. Treatment may include administering cholestyramine which binds to ochratoxin A and moves it to the intestines for elimination.

ACCIDENTS 161,374

Accidents are the number 1 killer for 0 – 44-year-olds and number 3 for 45 – 64. If it wasn't for chronic illnesses this would be the top killer. Of all Accidents falls are the number 1 killer for 65 and older.

<u>ACCIDENT TRENDS</u>

Bicycle crash	1,000
Accidental gunshot	2,500 (under 25 years old)
Drowning	4,000 (children)
Pedestrians hit by car	6,200
Falls	36,000
Car accident	38,000
Accidental Poisoning	65,000 (many Fe vitamins)

Motor vehicle accidents account for 24% of all work-related deaths. This is about 1,250 deaths per year. It breaks down to 39% from semis, 13% from pick-up trucks, 10% from delivery trucks/vans and 10% from automobiles. This info is from the CDC.[43]

Drunk drivers are involved in 33% of traffic fatalities. Iowa is 4th in the nation for number of drunk drivers.[44]

Risky behaviors increase the likelihood of injury or death. Having an open mind and being willing to modify your behavior to be safe will reduce the potential for injuries. In addition to safer actions you can eat foods to make your body stronger and more resistant to injury.

1.)   VITAMIN K_2 – Increases bone density by removing calcium plaques from arteries & soft tissue & depositing the calcium in bones. This helps protect against injuries from falls.

2.)   BIKE HELMETS – Of the 1,000 annual deaths from bicycle crashes about 750 are from head injuries. Most bicycle accidents occur when it is dark; wear light colored clothing, ensure reflectors are clean and make use of a light.

3.)	DOWNTOWN – Avoid driving downtown, during rush hour or other busy times to reduce the incidence of accidents.

4.)	FIREARMS – If you have them keep them locked up. Store ammunition separately from weapons. Safety classes.

5.)	WORK a job that is not likely to incur life threatening accidents.

6.)	HYDROLYZED COLLAGEN – When eaten it increases bone density which helps protect against falls. Topical application of collage has been shown to have no effect on skin.

7.)	ALCOHOL - Avoid excessive alcohol and drugs.

8.)	GARLIC - Raw garlic. Offsets bone damage caused by smoking by protecting osteoblasts (which lay new bone matrix.) This makes for stronger bones. Elephant garlic is not garlic.

9.)	DRIVE a safe vehicle, not a cool vehicle.

10.)	LEARN TO SWIM. Teach your children to swim even at a young age. Pay for swim lessons for grandchildren. Offer to take them to the lessons if the parents cannot. Pay for others to take lessons like a grant or set up a program. Drowning makes up about 4,000 deaths annually. 90% of parents whose child drowns end up getting a divorce. Drowning is more dangerous than firearms. Swim with your young children to acclimate them to being in the water.

11.)	OMEGA 3 FATTY ACID – Low omega 3 fatty acid content of brains is correlated with those who commit suicide.

12.)	DROWSY DRIVING – More people die from accidents attributed to drowsy driving than from drunk driving.

13.)	MAGNETIC STIMULATION – A coil of wire with an electric current is used to stimulate muscles and nerves. Used to speed up wound healing in muscles, connective tissues and nerves. Appears to work by exercising muscles without actually performing exercise. Has many other positive benefits too. *"The thighs of the animals were placed at the center of the coil, and each MS session was performed as described previously (10 min/10Hz and 10min/50 Hz, each pulse consisting of 3 s stimulation, 6 s rest)."*[45] A new device demonstrating better results involves placing the injured body part in a tube and applying static magnetic field. The tube may be using a Helmholtz Coil or Maxwell Coil. Also, Pulsed Electromagnetic Field therapy (PEMF).

14.)   DANGEROUS INTERSECTIONS – Many states and sometimes cities maintain a list of their most dangerous intersections. Avoid these during busy times or when there is construction.

Central IOWA[46]

City	Intersection	Accidents	Deaths
Ankeny	N. Ankeny Blvd & 1st St.	57	0
DSM	Day St. & 6th Ave.	55	1
DSM	E. 30th & University	73	0
Ankeny	Ankeny Blvd & SE Magazine	38	1
Ankeny	S. Ankeny Blvd & SW 3rd	62	0
DSM	E. Euclid & E. 14th St.	83	0
Ankeny	SW Oralabor & SW State St.	96	0
DSM	E. Army Post & S.E. 5th St.	50	1
DSM	SE 5th & Indianola & SE 6th	44	0
Polk Co.	NE 78th & NE 56th	14	1
WDM	1st/63rd & Railroad		
WDM	1st/63rd & Grand		
WDM	Vista & Jordan Creek Parkway		

Another resource for Iowans is a crash mapping tool.[47]

15.)   CROSSING THE STREET – As a pedestrian look up from your phone when crossing the street and look both ways. The Governor's Highway Safety Commission reported over 6,000 pedestrian deaths last year. Collecting data on why a pedestrian was hit is difficult to measure. Many of these people never looked up from their phones.

16.)   IMPROVE BALANCE – Exercise to improve your balance to reduce fall incidence. You can work on stretches or balancing, but for extra credit try the brain dance.

17.)   SEAT BELT MODIFICATION – It's difficult to improve upon the 3-point system in most vehicles. The 5-point harness used in baby seats and NASCAR should not be carried over to the standard seatbelt system in your vehicle. 5-point harnesses have been tested and studied for their specific applications and shown to provide increased safety only in those situations. Same thing goes for the 3-point seatbelt in your vehicle. Adding a seatbelt pad to soften the blow from a crash has shown an increase in fatalities by ejecting the user from the vehicle. This may be because the body rolls the pad around the seatbelt reducing its ability to secure the body. In a crash this results in the body sliding out of the seatbelt.

18.)   RECALLS – The National Highway Traffic Safety Administration manages and issues recalls for automotive vehicles in the United States. Recalls are only issued for safety reasons. Search their website by your vehicle's VIN.[48] If your vehicle has a recall contact your dealer to see if they have a record of it already being serviced. If not, then get it fixed.

The VIN is like a social security number for vehicles. It stands for Vehicle Identification Number and is unique to every vehicle. You may find your vehicle's VIN by looking at the windshield from the outside. Look at the bottom on the driver's side. It should also be on your insurance policy and title to the vehicle and vehicle registration.

The NHTSA also issues recalls for tires. The same website tracks this information.

19.)   CRIME – You can check crimemaping.com to see the crimes in your area. This can be useful for determining where to live, where to shop, vacation planning, etc. Not all communities report to this database.

The CDC tracks homicides. In 2017 about 19,000 people were murdered. 7 of the top 10 states are in the south.

20.)   SODIUM – Increase sodium consumption to prevent dizziness upon standing up.

RESPIRATORY DISEASE 154,596
CHRONIC LOWER (asthma, COPD, pulmonary

hypertension)

1.)   DON'T SMOKE - If you are pregnant and smoke then take 500mg of vitamin C or more each day. Smoking increases oxidation. Vitamin C is an antioxidant able to negate a lot of the harm caused by nicotine to your unborn child. Doing this can reduce newborn deaths.[49]

2.)   INDOOR AIR POLLUTION – Clean, dust, disinfect and vacuum frequently. Wash bedding frequently. Open windows. Place cat litter in space not used and use a litter box with a lid.

A.) Carbon Monoxide – Use a carbon monoxide detector. Common sources of CO_2 are smoking, defective furnace, defective water heater and car exhaust.

B.) Volatile Organic Compounds - Chlorinated water – Heated chlorine turns into chloroform which is highly toxic. Use of chlorine filters in showers and baths is most effective. Faucet filters exist too. Use cold or cooler temp showers.

C.) Furnace Filter – Replace the furnace filter sooner than recommended. Get only high-quality filters. Some have activated carbon to filter out smoke and other odors.

D.) Indoor Ventilation – Poor ventilation causes accumulation of compounds like carbon dioxide. Open windows and doors in warm weather.

E.) Organic Mattress – Most mattress manufacturers cover new furniture with toxic chemicals to make them resistant to fire. Remember opening a new mattress? That smell is from all those chemicals escaping from the fabric and getting into the air. These chemicals are also applied to baby clothes and car fabric. Organic mattresses do not have these chemicals.

F.) UVC Light – Ultraviolet C light is produced by the sun just like UVA, UVB, visible light, etc., but it is filtered out by the atmosphere before it reaches the Earth's surface. UVC light is highly toxic and will kill just about anything it touches. You can order a UVC light bulb from Amazon and plug it into any lamp or light fixture. Be careful as it will cause cancer if it reaches your skin and it will make plastic and rubber deteriorate.

3.)   HYGEINE HYPOTHESIS – Children raised in extremely clean environments tend to develop a variety of allergies and asthma. Children allowed to get dirty tend to develop less of an incidence of allergies and asthma. Having a household pet, visiting petting zoos, zoos or farm animals are all ways to expose your child to a host of dirt and germs in a good way.

There is an inverse relationship in children who have *Helicobacter pylori* in their stomachs and the presence of asthma. In other words, kids who do not have *H. pylori* in their stomachs also develop asthma.[50] The point being that sometimes harmful microbes are associated with a benefit. Perhaps this has to do with a commensal balance with other microbes which would be negatively impacted by a very clean environment.

4.)   LYCOPENE – 30mg/day decreased exercise induced asthma. The study does not state if the lycopene was consumed with fat. Lycopene is a fat-soluble molecule. It's ability to be absorbed by the GI tract increases from almost 0 to therapeutic amounts when fat is ingested at the same time. It also works better when taken with tomato products.[51]

5.)   POLLUTION – Pollution induced asthma is significantly more common in urban areas than rural areas. Citylab has an interactive map[52] that breaks down each county in America and lists the data that went into it.

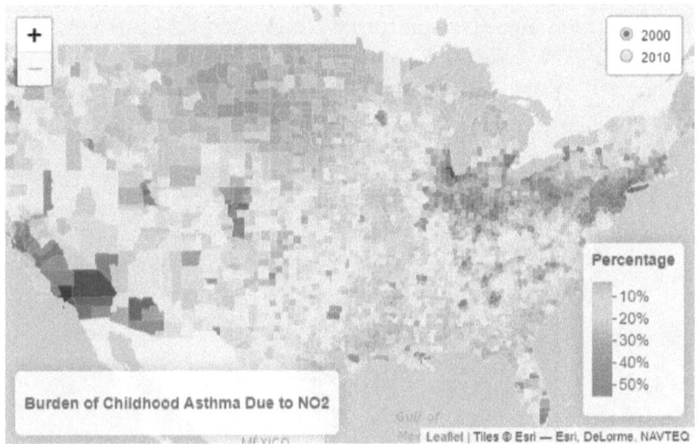

There are several online trackers for up-to-date air quality status. AirNow[53] is an easy to use one.

In the 1990's California initiated efforts to improve air quality. A well-designed study showed that reducing nitrogen dioxide and particulate matter also decreased rates of childhood asthma.[54]

6.)   MUCO-CILLIATED STATE – A newly discovered asthmatic cell line contributor decreases communication between cells in asthmatics. Dubbed the muco-cilliated state they increase inflammatory Th2 cells[55]. This is something to keep an eye on for future research.

7.)   BILIVERDIN – Heme breaks down into biliverdin. Biliverdin quickly breaks down into bilirubin. Biliverdin is a potent antioxidant, but because it breaks down into bilirubin so quickly it has very little chance of exerting any health benefits.

In a case report, "We report a case of complete resolution of persistent difficult-to-control asthma in accordance with increased levels of serum bilirubin due to acute hepatitis B." The hepatitis B caused hyperbilirubinemia which manifested as jaundice. The authors state the unknown cause for the remission of asthma, but theorize that it has to do with hyperbilirubinemia.[56] Biliverdin levels would have to be higher in order to increase bilirubin levels.

8.)   MICROBIOME – Changes in the microbiome take place during asthma flare ups and then return to a different state once it is over. The flair ups are associated with *Staphylococcus, Streptococcus* and *Moraxella* species. Periods of normal health are more associated with *Corynebacterium* and *Dolosigranulum*.[57] Further inquiry is needed to see if these strains can be altered to maintain the desired populations.

ALZHEIMERS 116,103, DEMENTIA & COGNITIVE DECLINE

In the last few years there have been some exciting discoveries involving Alzheimer's Disease and Dementia. These are:

1.) Discovery of the lymph system in the brain called the glymphatic system
2.) Roll of blood-brain barrier breakdown
3.) Gum disease is a likely cause
4.) The increasing probability that HSV-1 is another cause
5.) Amyloid and tau proteins cause other proteins to become harmful.

In all likelihood Alzheimer's Disease has many causes. This is why it has been so hard to find *the* cause. If you have a great glymphatic system you can clear toxic waste from your brain easily, but if you get terrible gum disease you may create too many toxins that overload your great waste removal system and end up with Alzheimer's. This could confuse researchers who may see that your gum disease doesn't match others who also have Alzheimer's, but have fantastic oral health. Further, someone else with an even better functioning glymphatic system may have the same gum disease you have, but be able to clear out the toxins produced by the infectious agent.

A microbe that causes periodontal disease creates enzymes that reach the brain and modify proteins which cause beta amyloid plaques and tau protein problems. Those with Alzheimer's Disease frequently have gum disease as well.

A breakdown in the blood-brain barrier allows these enzymes and other harmful toxins such as fibrinogen to enter the brain. Fibrinogen is needed to clot blood, but it should not pass the blood-brain barrier. Additionally, the importance of maintaining a proper blood sugar level is gaining a wider audience. Alzheimer's is increasingly being thought of as Type III Diabetes; meaning high blood sugar damages the brain.

When treated with antiviral medication used for HSV-1 and varicella zoster patients have been shown to delay the progression of dementia. Those infected who are not treated develop dementia sooner and progress worse at a faster rate.

If the glymphatic system is not functioning properly the brain is unable to clean out any harmful substances. This results in an accumulation of toxic substances.

The more amyloid plaque and tau present in the brain the more they will reproduce causing other proteins to misbehave.[58]

Hopefully, it's easy to see that there are likely multiple causes for cognitive decline; each may act independently or alongside other causes complicating the situation. There may be more causes that have not been identified. A 2017 review determined that dementia was an underlying cause in the deaths of over 261,000 people.[59] If this sort of cognitive decline is not the cause of death it is frequently a comorbid condition.

Based on these recent discoveries, in order to prevent Alzheimer's Disease, dementia and other brain disorders it would be best to incorporate practices which prevent or treat gum disease, ensure the health and repair of the blood-brain barrier, improve the functioning of the glymphatic system and treat or prevent HSV-1 and varicella infection. Other options are included below, however, the specifics to how these work are not always known, but it is likely that they improve something in the big 4 mentioned above.

1.)   CHOLESTEROL – Your brain needs cholesterol to function properly. Avoid cholesterol lowering drugs. Heart disease treatments became popular in the 1960's. Cholesterol lowering drugs were one of the popular treatments. 20 – 30 years later people who had been on cholesterol lowering drugs started getting diseases which impair brain function. They have been starving their brains for decades. Amyotrophic Lateral Sclerosis (ALS) is an example of a disease that is most likely caused by cholesterol lowering drugs. Most, but not all, of those with ALS have a long history of taking cholesterol lowering drugs.

Your body makes its own cholesterol from saturated fat. Ensure you eat enough saturated fat. Good sources are coconut oil, butter, and red meat.

A new theory of Alzheimer's Disease is that it involves cholesterol transport breakdown. This alters cholesterol distribution on a cell's surface negatively leading to neurodegeneration.[60] However, this study is behind a paywall. A review of the article[61] mentions cholesterol as the culprit behind Alzheimer's Disease and heart disease, but what it reports about the study does not match this conclusion. The issue is cholesterol transport, not cholesterol itself.

For those who sincerely wish to prevent or reverse Alzheimer's Disease please read Dale Bredesen's book The End of Alzheimer's.

2.)   (-) – EPICATECHIN – Found in raw chocolate, dramatically improves memory.

3.)   a – PINENE – Improves memory. Found in conifers and can be inhaled while walking through a conifer forest. Also present in rosemary oil.

4.)   CREATINE – Increases memory recall in vegetarians because they don't get any from their diet. May also help non-vegetarians if they don't eat much of it either. May improve dream recall.

5.)   HEALTHY FATS – DHA, other omega 3 oils and essential fatty acids, butter, coconut oil, olive oil, saturated fat, all help your brain function better. Most tissues of your body are comprised of water. Your brain, however, is mostly fat. If you have a low-fat diet expect to encounter problems with your brain function.

6.)   DIABETES – Having diabetes doubles the likelihood of developing dementia. Chronically elevated blood sugar levels damage proteins creating advanced glycation end products (AGEs) which cause oxidative damage and inflammation. They also contribute to the formation of and transportation across the blood-brain barrier of neurofibrillary tangles and amyloid beta plaques which are part of Alzheimer's. If that wasn't enough, chronically elevated insulin levels contribute to the formation of neurofibrillary tangles and amyloid plaques and decrease the function of the blood-brain barrier and contribute to strokes.

7.)   DIABETES – Insulin is not needed for glucose to cross the blood-brain barrier or to enter neurons. Chronically elevated blood glucose levels may negatively impact the way neurons metabolize glucose by inhibiting the brain's ability to utilize glycolysis to obtain energy. The glucose transporter protein GLUT3 is less active in those with Alzheimer's than in controls.

8.) TURMERIC – Growing evidence shows the curcumin in turmeric helps the brain function normally. Ingesting small amounts of curcumin over a period of several months can reduce signs of Alzheimer's and dementia. Turmeric increases the activity of enzymes that convert omega 3 fatty acid ALA into EPA and then DHA. However, DHA supplementation has not been shown to benefit those who already have Alzheimer's.

9.) EXERCISE – Older people who are physically fit have a reduced risk for dementia and Alzheimer's.[62, 63, 64, 65, 66]

10.) DEPRESSION – DHA – Hippocampus has shrunk in almost every person with depression. The hippocampus is one of only 2 areas of the brain that can grow new neurons and increase in size. 2g of DHA per day for 12 months significantly increased the size of the hippocampus and cerebrum and improved scores of those who have mild cognitive impairment.[67]

11.) GAMMA WAVES – Flickering lights at 40Hz (or gamma wavelengths of 25-140Hz) prevented and reversed amyloid plaque buildup and tau protein in the visual cortex of mice. Noise played at 40 Hz reduced amyloid plaque in hippocampus. Hippocampus sits closer to the auditory cortex than the visual cortex. Researchers saw increased activity in microglia. Microglia are the immune cells of the brain. They clean up the amyloid plaques and tau proteins. Alzheimer's patients have reduced gamma waves. The thought is that by inducing gamma waves in the brain microglia will become more active at cleaning up waste.[68] Caution as gamma oscillations can induce seizers. Note, that in the article the authors think auditory stimulus to be more effective than visual because the part of the brain, hippocampus, experiencing problems is closer to the part of the brain processing sound. This is in a mouse brain. If the visual processing part of a mouse brain is too far away to impact the hippocampus then neither of these treatments are likely to cover 100x the distance in a human brain.

12.)   SPIRULINA – Protects stem cells in the hippocampus and promotes their proliferation.[69] The hippocampus stores memories.

13.)   EXERCISE – Highly fit women in their 40's are 90% less likely to develop dementia than unfit women in their 40's. Of those fit women who develop dementia it is around age 90 which is 11 years later than less fit women. Initial fitness was assessed by a 6-minute bike ride. Those who biked the hardest were the most fit. Those who could not finish were unfit.[70]

14.)   EXTENDED SITTING – Sitting for long periods of time is associated with atrophy of the medial temporal lobe; a region of the brain that helps make new memories. Physical activity did not compensate for extended sitting periods. The sitting periods need to be interrupted.[71]

15.)   COFFEE – In mouse models, caffeine works synergistically with eicosanoyl-5-hydroxytryptamide which enhances enzyme action of phosphatase PP2A which breaks down a pathogenic protein called α-synuclein. PP2A does not work well in people with α-synucleinopathies which includes Parkinson's Disease and dementia with Lewy bodies.[72]

16.)   ALCOHOL – Low doses of alcohol help cerebrospinal fluid flush toxic substances out of the brain. High doses show no benefit and too much impairs the ability of cerebrospinal fluid of doing its job. The research on mice corresponds strongly with Blue Zones longevity research on humans.[73] The mice study equates to about 2.5 servings where 1 serving is 5 ounces of 12 percent wine or 12 ounces of 5 percent beer for 155 lbs person.[74]

17.)   OMEGA 3 FATTY ACIDS – Promote glymphatic system function. They promote amyloid-β clearance from the brain via the glymphatic system.[75]

18.)   BLOOD BRAIN BARRIER – The integrity of the blood-brain barrier falters before cognitive abilities with Alzheimer's. *"Our data show that individuals with early cognitive dysfunction develop brain capillary damage and BBB breakdown in the hippocampus irrespective of Alzheimer's Aβ and/or tau biomarker changes, suggesting that BBB breakdown is an early biomarker of human cognitive dysfunction independent of Aβ and tau."*[76]

Fibrinogen is a clotting factor used to repair holes in blood vessels. It is not present in the brain. Another study[77] showed that if the blood-brain barrier is impaired fibrinogen can cross into the brain causing immune cells to attack it and neurons destroying them. This destruction of synapses can lead to cognitive decline.

19.)   *Porphyromonas gingivalis* – A fairly new concept in Alzheimer's Disease progression is that this microbe responsible for chronic periodontitis is also the culprit in Alzheimer's Disease. Gingipains are toxic proteases (a protease is an enzyme that breaks down proteins) created by *P. gingivalis*. Mice with *P.* gingivalis infection showed increased amounts of amyloid plaques and had detrimental effects on tau protein. Beyond this correlation, to further demonstrate gingipains as the source of the problem, researchers created a gingipain inhibitor which was able to reduce its effects on those with *P. gingivalis* infection. This was established by showing a decrease in amyloid beta plaque production, neuroinflammation and rescued neurons in the hippocampus.[78] Most of these were shown in mice models.

20.)   HSV-1 – More commonly known as the cold sore virus. An infection is lifelong. When not active the virus retreats to a nerve leading to the brain. Those treated with antivirals are significantly less likely to develop dementia than those who aren't treated.[79] In addition to this, viruses alter their nearby surroundings. They end up developing what's called a protein corona along the outside of themselves. They can denature proteins they come into contact with causing them to behave in ways they aren't supposed to.[80] This impacts not just Alzheimer's Disease, but also other brain disease such as Parkinson's Disease.

21.)   WALNUTS – Consumption of walnuts provides a host of benefits to the brain. Taken from the abstract, *"walnuts not only reduce the oxidant and inflammatory load on brain cells but also improve interneuronal signaling, increase neurogenesis, and enhance sequestration of insoluble toxic protein aggregates.*"[81] Walnuts contain a lot of nutrients that have been studied and shown to have benefits to health, mostly to the brain.

22.)   IRISIN – The precursor is FNDC5 (Fibronectin type III domain-containing protein 5). Discovered in the 2000's, Irisin is a hormone produced when muscles contract. Exercise dramatically increases production. A study[82] in January 2019 found that irisin also promotes neurogenesis of the hippocampus. Those with Alzheimer's Disease have significantly lower amounts of irisin in the hippocampus, mice treated to increase irisin levels *"rescued synaptic plasticity and memory in AD mouse models,"* knockout mice with lower irisin levels have worse memory than controls. The takeaway here is that exercise increases irisin levels which protect and heal the hippocampus where long term memories are stored and likely plays a part in preventing Alzheimer's Disease.

23.)   CHOLESTEROL – Your brain requires cholesterol to function properly. Without it your neurons wither and die.

24.)   DHA – It is unlikely that DHA will reverse symptoms of someone who has been diagnosed with Alzheimer's Disease; however, it has been shown that DHA markedly increases the activity of an enzyme, LR11, responsible for clearing away amyloid plaques. Increasing levels of DHA increase LR11.[83]

25.)   tACS – Transcration Alternating Current Stimulation alters theta brainwaves of the hippocampus which improves working memory in those with impaired memory.[84]

26.)   0.75Hz WAVE INDUCTION – Applying 0.75Hz waves to the hippocampus during Non-REM sleep enhances declarative memory retention of the hippocampus.[85] This might be because those who benefit have weakened electrical waves to begin with. Application of the 0.75Hz waves might provide a boost to those who are low.

27.)   LACK OF DEEP SLEEP – Failure to move through each phase of sleep for the required amount of time increases β-amyloid retention in the brain by preventing the ability of cerebrospinal fluid from flushing it out.[86]

It should be noted that almost every sleep medication induces *sedation* not sleep. Sleep pills prevent the brain's ability to move through the normal stages of sleep. Simply being unconscious is not the same as sleeping.

28.)   TRAUMATIC BRAIN INJURY – Any sort of brain damage significantly increases the likelihood of developing Alzheimer's Disease. If you have an Apeo4 allele you are even more likely to develop it after an injury. Lactate or BHB (butyrate) may prevent the effects of traumatic brain injury.

29.)   ANTICHOLINERGIC DRUGS – There exists a very strong association for increased rates of dementia and use of anticholinergic medication. Drugs that have anticholinergic effects are used in antidepressants, antiparkinsons disease, antipsychotics, bladder antimuscarinics and antiepileptics.[87]

30.)   CARBS BEFORE BED – Insulin Degrading Enzyme is responsible for breaking down insulin after insulin is finished transporting glucose. It has another function; that of breaking down amyloid. It cannot do both at the same time. By avoiding carbohydrates prior to bedtime you prevent insulin levels from rising. This frees up insulin degrading enzyme so that it can focus its attention on amyloid. Carbs before bed ensure insulin degrading enzyme will spend all of its time breaking down insulin which will allow amyloid to accumulate.

31.)   ELDERBERRY – Sambucus nigra has been show to prevent cold and flu viruses from replicating. (See #9 under Influenza and Pneumonia.) I haven't found any studies on other viruses, but the way elderberry works on cold and flu could also work on other viruses such as the ones associated with Alzheimer's Disease.

32.)   SILICON – Aluminum is not a nutrient and yet it is present in amyloid plaques. Silicon competes with aluminum for absorption. Soft water has less silicon and more aluminum that hard water.

DIABETES 80,058

Diabetes is most likely responsible for more deaths than this as it causes heart disease, stroke, cancer, accidents, kidney disease and many other conditions. I would bet dollars to pesos that if you have Type II diabetes you are also overweight. Most people with Type II diabetes could reverse it completely if they employed a little fortitude and personal discipline to permanently change their lifestyle. If they don't their death certificates will read that diabetes was an underlying cause.

The more sensitive you can be to insulin the healthier you will be. Insulin insensitivity is what causes health problems with diabetes. By being sensitive to insulin you will require less glucose in your blood and therefore in your diet to meet the needs of your body.

How many grams of carbohydrates over what time period does it take to make someone a Type II diabetic? Every Type II diabetic was diagnosed at one point in time, but they didn't get there suddenly by accident. It took a lot of work eating all those carbs. How many carbs did it take? What if they had eaten the same amount, but over 10 more years? If you eat 2,000 calories a day you eat 730,000 calories a year. If you are diagnosed at 50 you've eaten roughly, 35,000,000 calories.

Count your calories.

If you can spread that 35 million out over a few more years you will be much healthier.

1.)   INSULIN – Reduce sugar consumption and overall caloric intake; especially high glycemic index foods which increases the insulin response of the pancreas. When eating high glycemic index foods eat them with other foods or in a meal. Their glycemic index rating comes from testing each food individually; however, when one food is eaten with another the glycemic impacts change significantly.

2.)   EXERCISE – Cardio is best, resistance training such as lifting weights is also beneficial. Doing both is even better.

3.)   CALORIC RESTRICTION – Another way to think of this is to eat fewer calories than you burn. This results in weight loss. Type II Diabetes has often been considered a lifelong disease. However, it can be reversed immediately. *"In the first 7 days of the reduced energy intake, fasting blood glucose and hepatic insulin sensitivity fell to normal, and intrahepatic lipid decreased by 30%. Over the 8 weeks of dietary energy restriction, beta cell function increased towards normal and pancreatic fat decreased."*[88]

The main point of the study was to establish the fact that fat accumulation around the pancreas damages pancreas function. Removal of the fat allows the pancreas to return to normal. This was accomplished by eating less energy. In fact, the study only stated that the participants consumed less energy, but it never states what it is less than. Was it less than was previously consumed? Was it less energy/calories than they burned?

The full quote from above ends with a statement that the study participants actually gained weight after the 8 weeks was up. This leads me to believe they ate fewer calories than before resulting in a slower weight gain or they felt like they had less energy so they moved less which would result in burning fewer calories.

I've filed this under 'Caloric Restriction' because a diabetic consuming fewer calories than he burns will likely result in even greater benefits.

Another study found that after 3 months of about 1500 calories/day, 1 hour of brisk walking/day and metformin, 53% of study participants completely reversed their diabetes while another 22% partially reversed it. The study followed them for 2 years where rates of complete reversal were 47% and partial reversal were 22%.[89]

4.)   PTEROSTILBENE – A nutrient found in many foods; mostly in the Vaccinium family. It reduces reactive oxygen species, overproduction of human retinal endothelial cells, TNF α, IL-β, and NF-$\varkappa$B protein. All of this means it can delay the progression of diabetic retinopathy.[90]

5.)   POOR SLEEP – Not sleeping well causes β cells of the pancreas to be less sensitive to blood glucose resulting in releasing less insulin. Further, poor sleep causes a significant 30% reduction in a cell's ability to respond to insulin. This means consumption of just a little sugar will result in an elevated blood glucose level which will remain elevated longer.[91] Elevated blood glucose levels lead to a host of other fatal illnesses some of which are the leading causes of death mentioned in this notebook.

6.)   COW MILK – The main protein in milk is casein, but it has different forms. Casein A1 is in cow milk. Casein A2 is present in goat milk and almost every other animal. *"Previously, two potential pathways have been suggested as being involved in the link between type 1 diabetes and A1 β-casein: (i) the opioid activity of BCM-7;54 and (ii) the similar structures of β-casein and an epitope of the glucose transporter 2 (GLUT-2) expressed on β-cells (that is, immunological cross-reactivity or molecular mimicry)."*[92] Some people think that casein A1 contributes to the development of diabetes

7.)   SODIUM – As stated under #21 in Heart Disease and Stroke, most people naturally eat about 3-4 grams of sodium per day. The kidneys regulate sodium and when you reduce sodium intake under what is needed they create renin, angiotensin and aldosterone. These hormones cause the body to retain salt. They also cause insulin levels to increase. The longer you are on a low salt diet the more likely you are to have chronic elevated insulin levels despite healthy carbohydrate intake. In short, sodium improves the body's ability to use glucose.

INFLUENZA & PNEUMONIA 12,000 – 79,000

The flu is the one infectious disease in the top 10. It kills thousands of people every year and usually peaks around January to February. In a typical year it mostly kills those who are vulnerable with weakened immune systems; the elderly and newborns. However, when the flu is extra deadly it tends to kill those who are generally considered healthy and not those with weakened immune systems. There is no adequate explanation for this.

The 2017-2018 flu season was one of the worst on record. Almost 80,000 Americans died. The flu vaccine was largely ineffective.[93]

SEASON	DEATHS[94]
2017-2018	79,000
2016-2017	51,000
2015-2016	25,000
2014-2015	51,000
2013-2014	38,000
2012-2013	43,000
2011-2012	12,000
2010-2011	37,000

1.)   WASH HANDS – The no brainer of cleanliness. Hand sanitizer is probably not as effective at killing germs as washing hands with soap and water. If you are having a hard time preventing the flu you could try some other options for soap. Sulphur soap is made of something like 10% sulphur. It does not smell the best, but usually comes in a sealed jar. Sulphur is great at killing germs. Another option is salt soap. It isn't soap. It's a bar of salt about the size of a bar of soap. Salt is excellent at killing germs. In fact, nothing can live in pure salt environments. The salt bar also leaves your skin extra soft to the touch. Both can be purchased on Amazon for under $20.

2.)   VITAMIN C and ZINC – Low levels impair the function of the immune system.

3.)   OREGANO OIL – Orally ingested oregano oil could help fight infections.

4.)   COPPER SURFACES – Copper has the ability to kill microbes. Replace door knobs, faucet handles, etc. with copper ones to reduce the presence of microbes.

5.)   SOCIAL EXPOSURE – Limit contact with others during sick season especially you know they are sick. Avoid children's play places, doctor's offices, nurseries, etc.

6.)   DO YOUR PART – If you are sick stay away from others especially if they are vulnerable. Cough into your hands or arm.

7.)   IRON – High iron levels may reduce your ability to fight infections. This study was done on hemodialysis patients.[95]

8.)   tBHQ – tBHQ is a preservative added to many foods. It reduces the immune response by decreasing CD8 T cells in the lung and CD4 and CD8 T cells were unable to identify flu virus. It also reduced the ability of the immune system to remember the flu virus during a later infection.[96]

9.)   ELDERBERRY – Studies are on *Sambucus nigra L.* Elderberries have been shown to prevent the flu virus from entering a cell and stopping viral replication in its later stages.[97] Another study discovered the mechanism of action; two substances found in elderberries latch onto the virion - the virus before it enters the host cell - and prevent it from entering a cell to replicate. "*…that flavonoids from the elderberry extract bind to H1N1 virions and, when bound, block the ability of the viruses to infect host cells.*"[98]
Other studies demonstrate elderberry's effectiveness at reducing flu incidence and severity of symptoms. The authors concluded that travelers who consumed their elderberry extract experienced, "*…a significant reduction of cold duration and severity…*"[99]
Elderberry is currently being evaluated for safety.[100]
Would black elderberry be effective against other viruses?

10.)   FLU VACCINE – Some swear by it. Some don't. In the summer pharmaceutical companies look at the flu in Australia as it is winter there. They guess which strain will be the most common in America. Even if they guess right the way the flu vaccine is grown promotes mutations from the original strain. This means the final strain in the shot you get can be different than what was intended. If they happened to guess the right major flu strain, but the virus mutated the shot's effectiveness is undermined. This is what happened in the 2016-2017 flu season. They guessed right. The flu mutated. The shot was not effective.

There's also a dozen or more strains of flu for any given season. The flu shot does not attempt to address all of them.

The flu can be nasty and people can die from it, but if you implement other things to keep your immune system healthy you probably won't ever need a flu shot.

11.)   HIGH TEMPERATURE & HIGH HUMIDITY – Guinea pigs are incredibly susceptible to human influenza viruses. When sick guinea pigs are placed next to healthy ones the healthy ones get sick when the air is blown in from the cages of the sick ones. As the temperature and humidity increased the transmission of flu to the healthy guinea pigs decreased. Once the temperature reached 86°F the flu failed to infect any of the healthy guinea pigs.

In addition, there maybe a correlation to record cold winters and flu prevalence or even large outbreaks at least in temperate climates. The flu of 1889 that started in London may have been caused by extreme cold that year. The 1880's were very cold in the Midwest. I need to look into this further.

KIDNEY DISEASE 50,546

1.) ANALGESICS – Avoid analgesics because they cause kidney damage over long term use. Kidneys make the hormone prostaglandin E2 which regulates blood flow to the kidneys. NSAIDS inhibit prostaglandin E2 production which reduces blood flow to the kidneys. Cessation of NSAIDS often results in normal kidney function.

2.) ACIDIC FOODS - Acidic foods may contribute to kidney damage causing protein to leak out of the kidneys into the urine. Meat tends to be acidic while fruits, vegetables and grains may be protective.

3.) DIABETES – Diabetes can lead to kidney failure.

4.) BLOOD PRESSURE – High blood pressure leads to kidney disease.

5.) WATER CONSUMPTION – Increasing water consumption decreases long term reduction in kidney cyst growth and fibrosis. It even helped with genetic causes of kidney disease and decreased hypertension.[101]

6.) OCHRATOXIN A – See TESTICULAR CANCER.

7.) PROTEIN KINASE C-ALPHA INHIBITOR – This manmade antibody targets connective tissue that is unique to kidneys. It reduces inflammation and restores mitochondrial function which significantly improved kidney function.[102]

TRENDS

The following trends are things that I've noticed that aren't necessarily top 10 killers, but they may cause or exacerbate diseases. They are often looked at singularly and because of this they easily fly under the big picture radar; their relation to other disease is often overlooked.

This is a working list. It is perhaps the most difficult section to put together as it involves noticing seemingly unrelated topics and connecting them in a way that has not been done before.

Accidents

The average age of death in America is in the upper 70's. The cause is usually a self-induced chronic disease that has been getting worse for decades. If any changes are made to avoid these unnecessary ways of dying then the next area of concern should be accident avoidance as it is the leading cause of death for people ages 0 – 44 and the leading cause of death for every other age group other than the chronic diseases already mentioned.

Aging GI Tract

As you age your gastrointestinal tract deteriorates. This impairs its ability to consume, digest and absorb nutrients. The lack of nutrients leads to illness and death. This occurs with centenarians who have the same most common causes of death as the rest of the population. Their healthy lifestyle prolonged life, but only delayed the onset of fatal illness. The point here is that this deterioration in health is often the result of modifiable behaviors; behaviors which you can change to avoid the deterioration. These are listed below according to location in the GI tract.

A special note should be given for gut microbes. Decades of poor nutrition can alter the composition of gut microbes in a way that further causes poor nutrition. An aging GI tract can impact food choice which will also alter gut microbe populations.

ORAL CAVITY
Dysphagia – difficulty initiating swallowing to feel
      food get stuck in the throat. Acutely caused
      by stroke. Over time it is caused by

Parkinson's Disease, muscular dystrophy. Can also be caused by dehydration.

Dentures – A lifetime of neglecting the health of your teeth can result in removing them. Dentures are not a perfect fix as many times people don't take the time to put them in, they don't work right, aren't properly cleaned which leads to infection, aren't able to be used the same way as teeth, etc. All this leads to a significant alteration in diet and nutrient intake.

ESOPHAGUS

Lower esophageal sphincter hypertension.

Obstruction caused by tumor, enlarged aorta, enlarged lymph nodes, etc.

Painful swallowing resulting from mucosal disruptions caused by pill induced esophagitis. (Is this caused by swallowing too many large and hard pills?)

GERD often treated by proton pump inhibitors which are strongly linked to other diseases. Also, biphosphate and NSAID's can cause GERD. The stomach acid pumped up by GERD into the esophagus can, over time, cause esophageal cancer.

STOMACH

Peptic Ulcer

H. pylori infection

Gastric atrophy causes malabsorption of vitamin B12, folate, iron and calcium.

SMALL INTESTINE

Celiac Disease – 25% of diagnoses are in people older than 60.

Anemia – microlytic anemia causes low iron levels. Macrolytic anemia causes low vitamin B12 and low folate. Anemia is the 1st symptom of malabsorption of the GI tract.

Crohn's Disease, Celiac Disease and surgery cause vitamin B12 deficiency.

Chronic *H. pylori* infection, metformin, H2 blockers and proton pump inhibitors cause overgrowth and infection.

Diarrhea – Lower levels of anaerobes and Bifidobacterium and increased levels of enterobacterium can cause problems. These changes in microbiota are often observed in older people.

Malnutrition – Severe malnutrition causes the intestine to shrink dramatically. This can also be caused by a lack of vitamin D. Caloric restriction increases the amount of intestinal stem cells, but they don't do anything unless vitamin D is present.

LARGE INTESTINE

Diverticular Disease – NSAID's and opiates used by elderly can cause this. Also, lack of fiber.

Colo-rectal Cancer – 90% of diagnoses are in those older than 50.

All of the conditions listed above lead to decreased consumption, digestion and/or absorption of nutrients. As these conditions progress slowly over time the body's ability to function with lower levels of needed nutrients will be difficult to notice and likely be attributed to 'normal aging.' In reality, the body is suffering from lack of nutrition. For example, many centenarians have small red blood cells. This is likely caused by lack of iron. Low iron causes the body to make small red blood cells; a condition called microlytic anemia.

Most of the information from above was taken from one in depth study.[103]

Changes over time in microbiota of the GI tract result in a decrease in production and absorption of nutrients. Notably, carotenoids and polyphenols. Protein consumption directly impacts several hormones. Do dietary habits change over time resulting in less protein consumption? Eating less protein would prevent formation of many enzymes and hormones and would cause muscle atrophy. Cutting salt for many years will cause osteoporosis and diabetes.

Bottom Dwellers

Don't eat bottom dwellers. These are usually creatures that eat dead animals. Others are omnivores that tend to eat a variety of things which includes dead things. Some are filter feeders; they filter garbage out of the environment and concentrate toxins in their tissues. Examples include, pig, cod, crab, shrimp, snail, oyster, clam.

Centenarians

Centenarians die from the same causes as everyone else. The top 5 causes of death among those who live to 100 or older are:

1.) Heart Disease
2.) Alzheimer's
3.) Stroke
4.) Cancer
5.) Influenza and Pneumonia

This is from the CDC for 2016 published data. A study from 2005 confirms similar causes of death. It also showed that centenarians died with comorbidities and preexisting conditions. They were unhealthy for a long period of time.[104]

Another study shows that centenarians are usually born during September, October or November. Much speculation surrounds why this is the case. The same study lists several possible reasons why. It also states the Sep-Nov birth month has a strong presence in birth cohorts prior to 1900, but it disappears after this.[105]

One reason not mentioned by the study may have to do with the advent of home refrigeration. Those born Sep-Nov would be born shortly after harvest comes in. Their mothers would have a wider variety of fresh foods which would contribute to more nutritious breast milk. Those born in the Spring or Summer would have mothers whose food supply was less nutritious as the nutrients in preserved food deteriorate over time.

Home refrigeration became popular in the late 1920's. With it fresh fruits, vegetables, meat and dairy products could be preserved long term allowing mothers to eat more nutritious foods year round. This, in turn, would level out the overall health of children born at any time of the year.

Diet

Possible changes to diet as people age include, lower protein intake, lower sodium, lower fat especially saturated fat, lower silicon, increased carbohydrate. All of these are the opposite of what should happen.

Microbiome

Most of us are aware of probiotics for your gut, but microbes live almost everywhere in and on your body. You have a specific 'signature' of microbes for each part of your body. Certain healthy microbes are needed to maintain good health. Others can cause disease.

Manufacturers are making probiotic products for each of these areas. For example, the eye was previously thought to be sterile. The only microbes present were ones that temporarily contacted the eye and were quickly washed away. This has been discovered to not be true. There are 4 core genera of bacteria that are present in the eyes; *Staphylococci, Corynebacteria, Propionibacteria* and *Streptococci*.[106] There may be more. The composition present will vary depending on age, geography, ethnicity, use of contact lenses and type of contact lenses and disease presence.

In addition to the eye you also have a microbiome on your skin, sinuses and likely other places too. Supplementation with probiotics can help restore an imbalanced microbiome.

Prescription Drugs

128,000 people die every year from adverse reactions to prescription drugs.[107] This makes prescription drugs the 6th leading cause of death. This figure does not include intentional overdose or suicide.

Progeria – Accelerated aging. We all have progerin. Progerin is a protein that malfunctions as we age. Progerin binds to the Nrf2 protein so it can't work inside the nucleus. NAD+ treats progeria to a degree. NA Riboside increases NAD+. Do all humans have a form of progeria? If so, this means that what we perceive as normal aging is actually accelerated aging.

Sleep Deprivation

Lack of sleep causes every bodily system to worsen and fall apart; can test positive for diabetes, have heart attacks, develop cancer, develop psychosis, etc. Poor sleep is perhaps one of the largest contributors to chronic illness.

Hops can reverse the stimulating effects of caffeine. The neurotransmitter, adenosine, increases throughout the day causing drowsiness. Caffeine is an adenosine receptor antagonist meaning it binds to adenosine receptors on neurons and prevents them from being activated by adenosine. Studies show hops in combination with valerian negate the effects of caffeine[108], however, I've never noticed any benefit with valerian root; I have noticed this negating effect with only hops flowers or hops extract.

Transcutaneous Vagus Nerve Stimulation

As we age the sympathetic nervous system can become too active. This means there is an increase in the fight-or-flight response. There are various was to calm the sympathetic nervous system and increase activity of the parasympathetic nervous system. In the scientific world researchers place electrodes on a part of the ear lobe. The electric current stimulates the vagus nerve. Their word for this is called 'tickle therapy.' Another way to accomplish a similar result is to have your 'daith pierced.' Technically, this is a pierce in the anterior notch of the ear lobe.

Electrodes are considered effective; daith piercing is poo-pooed by medical experts even by those that treat migraines. In all likelihood, they both accomplish the same thing; the constant touch activates the nerve endings which travel along the vagus nerve to the brain.[109]

TRENDS IN ENDOTHELIUM CONCERNS

Blood-Brain Barrier

Breakdown in the blood-brain barrier allows toxins to enter the brain. This causes brain damage much earlier than previously thought and is now strongly associated with the development of memory loss, dementia and Alzheimer's Disease.

Glycation

May better be understood if considered under the chemistry term 'cross-link' as advanced glycation end products (AGE's) are formed by a cross-link. Formed when sugars are cooked with fats or proteins; grilled meat, caramelized food coloring, etc. Proteins and fats become glycated. These advanced glycation end products wreak havoc on many tissues; traps low density lipoprotein (LDL) cholesterol, causes collagen to stiffen vascular tissues, causes cataracts, muscle loss and contributes to Alzheimer's Disease. Diabetes can exacerbate advanced glycation end product formation as it greatly increases the amount of glucose available.

Some substances can reverse or prevent the negative effects of AGE's; vitamin C, alpha-lipoic acid, aspirin, carnosine, lycopene, resveratrol, curcumin and rosmarinic acid (from Rosemary) are a few easy to come by examples.[110] There are other substances as well.

Hardening of Soft Tissues

This is one of the largest issues with health in older people. Safe levels of many nutrients are not accurately established. Adhering to these levels may avoid instant death and prevent malnutrition, however, the safe ranges have not been updated to reflect safe upper limits. As it turns out people who have levels of various nutrients at the higher end of these safe levels develop, after years, serious health issues.

General strategies to reduce metal accumulation in soft tissues include, fasting, reducing calories and modifying diet to avoid the target metal. All these reduce the amount of metals absorbed by the GI tract. Potassium and magnesium appear to be relatively safe.

Copper, iron and zinc are closely related to Alzheimer's Disease, but in unclear ways. High levels of zinc appear to exacerbate Alzheimer's, but zinc supplementation also reduces it. Copper is easily oxidized, but shares a similar uncertain relationship. Iron is often not assessed properly. Most studies show Alzheimer's patients have normal iron levels; however, as you will read below, the normal iron range is too high. It could be that those with Alzheimer's have had iron levels in the high end of the healthy range for a long time.

Potassium and magnesium seem to be the only two metals the body needs that don't cause disease. The only way to have too much of either of these would be for some sort of unusual environmental exposure such as ingesting a lot of supplements. High levels of these can be caused by other factors, but in and of themselves they are not likely to occur.

ALUMINUM – Accumulates in the brain and is associated with some types of Alzheimer's Disease. Silicon, a nutrient, competes for absorption with aluminum and promotes its excretion. Some Alzheimer's patients even improve once they increase their silicon consumptions. You need about 10mg a day 9 months.

CALCIUM – Calcification of soft tissues can be caused by too much dietary calcium, too little vitamin K_2. Increasing levels of calcified soft tissue is considered normal in America, however, this is based on observational data, not on health. Calcium can be measured directly in the blood or urine.

      Decrease calcium consumption.
      Increase vitamin K_2.
      Increase magnesium.

COPPER – Maintain a copper:zinc ratio of 1:8. Otherwise copper accumulates in soft tissues causing many problems as it is used in over 300 reactions in the body. Skin, fat digestion and neurological problems are common.

FAT – Not a metal, obviously, but worthy of inclusion here. Over time, as organs fail fat cells replace organ specific cells. For example, fat cells replace neurons in gray matter in the brain, liver cells, bone cells, etc. A 40-year-old man has the same sized legs as a teenager, but half the muscle. The muscle has been replaced by fat.

IRON – Hemochromatosis and blood transfusions can lead to iron overload. Excess iron is stored in the liver, pancreas causing diabetes, brain reducing cognitive function and other organs causing them to shut down. It causes problems in many other tissues. Also, causes joint pain and is deposited in the skin making it darker. High iron levels, maybe even within what is considered the normal range, over a lifetime may cause the problems mentioned. Centenarians often have lower than normal iron levels.

To understand your iron level you must measure your ferritin. Ferritin is an iron transport molecule within a cell. Typically accepted normal levels are form 20-500ng/dL. However, those who have 200ng/dL have high incidence of diseases. Those with 300ng/dL have even higher incidence of the same diseases. The trend continues all the way through the healthy ranges. Generally speaking, ferritin levels should be maintained under 90ng/dL. Please note that this figure is not firmly established. The wide range may reflect that serum ferritin is not regulated by the body. Since ferritin is only used within a cell its presence in serum may be more indicative of its leakage and therefor represent a state of cellular damage or disease.[111]

Neuromelanin is produced by cells in the substantia nigra to protect themselves from oxidation. Iron is a major oxidizing agent of the substantia nigra in those with Parkinson's Disease.[112]

Yerba santa, *Eriodictyon californicum*, contains a substance called sterubin which has the ability to remove iron form neurons. Also, yerba santa contains eriodictyol, which has the same properties, but to a lesser extent. Sterubin has a host of other benefits for the brain. Studies[113] from the Salk Institute identified the presence of these substances in yerba santa and tested them. The focus of the study is on their technique to identify molecules with properties they have targeted; however, the targeted and tested ones show benefits to the brain.

The following strategies can be used to remove iron from the body or prevent iron accumulation.

REMOVAL
Blood donation/phlebotomy
Iron chelation therapy
Curcumin –
EGCG – Extract found in green tea. It crosses the blood brain barrier and is used to treat Alzheimer's Disease and prostate cancer.

Inositol Hexaphosphate (IP$_6$) – Cheap supplement. Treats Parkinson's Disease and many cancers.

Theaflavin – Extract found in black tea.

Quercetin – Crosses the blood brain barrier. Amount in food is not sufficient to reach therapeutic levels. You must use supplements.

Yerba santa

PREVENT ABSORPTION
Chocolate –
Coffee –
Eggs –
Dairy –
Grains and Vegetables –
Olive Oil –
Phytates (walnuts, almonds and legumes)
Red Wine –
Tea –

DECREASE IRON CONSUMPTION
Foods that increase iron absorption include: *Alcohol 25%, cast iron cooking, sugar* and *vitamin C.*

MAGNESIUM – Unlikely to have too much. Reduces calcification by binding with calcium in bones. Kidneys are very efficient at processing magnesium. Kidney disease or too many antacids with magnesium are the main causes of too much magnesium.

MANGANESE – Does not seem likely that you would be able to consume enough manganese to cause toxicity. However, there are several environmental sources that can and do cause toxicity: welding materials, car exhaust, pesticides, tap water and well water.

Symptoms are mostly neurological. It is often misdiagnosed as ALS (Lou Gehrig's Disease) or Parkinson's Disease.

Chelation therapy might help, but is not promising.

POTASSIUM – Not usually a problem. Symptoms can come from kidney problems, dehydration or too many potassium supplements or angiotensin II receptor blockers.

SELENIUM – Dietary toxicity does not seem to be common.

ZINC – Maintain a copper:zinc ratio of 1:8. Most of the time hyperzincemia manifests as having too little copper as zinc decreases copper absorption. Denture glue has enough zinc to cause hyperzincemia. The body has 2-3g of zinc. 90% of it is in muscles and bones. The rest is in the prostate, GI tract, kidney, skin, lung, brain and pancreas.

High doses lower the function of the immune system. Free zinc is a neurotransmitter. Zinc accumulates in dead and dying neurons[114].

The hippocampus is the first region of the brain to fail in Alzheimer's Disease. Zinc causes fibrinogen to clot. Zinc levels increase in the hippocampus in those with Alzheimer's Disease while their serum levels are normal.[115]

None of this means high levels of dietary zinc are a problem. Zinc storage, transport, etc. may result in dysfunction with how your body uses zinc.

Hypertension

Accepted knowledge is that as we age blood pressure gradually increases. Observed increases are about 1.5 mmHg for kids and 0.6 mmHg per year for adults. Ye'kuana people with limited western diets show an increase of 0.25 mmHg per year. Their neighbors, the Yanomami tribe, who have not adopted any western practices show 0 changes in blood pressure from childhood through old age.

Yanomami	95 over 63
American adult	121 over 71

The researchers attributed the healthy blood pressure to a better lifelong diet.[116] However, lifestyle differences likely account for this too. Things like exercise, time spent sedentary and sunshine impact overall health.

Elevated glucose levels, as found in diabetics, causes endothelial damage and hypertension.

Caffeine can elevate blood pressure 3-15mm/Hg over 4-13mm/Hg for 2 hours.[117]

An afternoon nap has been shown to lower blood pressure. The positive effects linger into the next day.[118]

Intestinal Endothelium

Fiber is food for microbes in the intestine. The mucus lining the inside of your intestines is made of a carbohydrate called mucin. Depriving these microbes of fiber causes them to consume mucin and pathogenic colonic microbes migrate to the small intestine where carbohydrates have not yet been digested and absorbed. The immune system then intervenes and can overreact causing problems.

Lead Poisoning

It has recently been discovered that lead poisoning is more common than realized as previously thought safe levels are only for acute lead poisoning. Safe levels of lead have been revised to lower figures several times over the last few decades. Lead levels in the blood in amounts far below what was thought to be safe now show accumulative impacts on the body especially blood vessel health. There is no safe level of lead in the blood. Lead is so damaging that it is now believed lower levels could be considered one of the top causes of death in the United States with over 400,000 deaths attributed to lead poisoning.

Avoid lead exposure.

Chelation therapy can remove lead.

EASY CHANGES

You just read a lot of information. It's a lot to digest. You may be overwhelmed with all those choices and changes into your lifestyle. I sure don't do everything I've written about to be healthy. Sometimes I just want to enjoy life and not think about how every action or inaction may or may not result in me dying early. Chowing down half a bag of potato chips sounds good to me any day.

To make life simpler let's consolidate a few things. In the list below I've gathered the most beneficial and easiest to adopt methods to improve your health.

1.) Drink more water - $0
2.) Better sleep habits - $0
3.) Get your ferritin level tested and reduce iron if need be - $0 if covered by insurance. $28 for a ferritin test from lifeextension.com.
4.) Get some sunlight - $0
5.) Get some cardio - $0
6.) Reach a healthy body weight - $0
7.) Eat a handful of walnuts everyday - $0.25/day
8.) Drink a little alcohol regularly - $1.00/day
9.) Eat lycopene preferably with tomato products and fat - $0.10/day
10.) Treat your cold sore with an antiviral - $0 if covered by insurance
11.) Eat omega 3's - $0.25/day
12.) Eat turmeric - $0.05/day
13.) Drink coffee or tea - $0 at work, church, etc. Otherwise $0.10/day at home.
14.) Take a cold shower - $0
15.) Donate blood - $0 + you save lives.
16.) Take a nap - $0
17.) Bone broth - $0 if you save your scraps.
18.) Eat 2 tablespoons of coconut oil every day.
19.) Eat more fat-soluble vitamins – A, D, E, K.

As you can see most of these are free. The most expensive item is $1.00 a day for a glass of $3.00 wine. The grand total is about $1.75 per day. This list is easy! Getting healthy and living a long healthy life is easy.

Pick 2 things from the list and start them today.

Next week add 2 more things.

Continue doing this for 4 weeks. If you want to keep going keep going. If not then get comfortable with the 8 healthy habits you've adopted into your life.

NEXT STEPS

If those best practices aren't enough for you then here are some suggestions to take it to the next level. The value with most of these is that you get hard to find phytonutrients not just vitamins and minerals.

1.) Homemade Bone Broth – A 10-pound bag of chicken quarters cost about $5. Cook these as usual, but save everything you don't eat. Put the bones, skin and everything else in the freezer. Save all other bones from other meals. Think steaks, ribs, pork shoulders; there's a ton of cuts of meat that leave the bone in. I highly recommend buying bones with marrow in them. A grocery store near me sells beef marrow bones for $8. Meat lockers will give you tons of bones also.

Put everything in a pressure cooker or instantpot. Cover with water. You can add vegetables if you like, but I don't. If you want the nutrients from the vegetables just eat them. I cook my broth for 90 minutes, release the steam and transfer the broth with some of the bones into a pot to reduce down a little. While it is reducing I fill the pressure cooker with new water and cook the same bones again for another 90 minutes. Once this batch is done I strain what is reducing and place in containers. Then I transfer all the bones and skin and everything in the instantpot into the large pot and reduce this batch down for 90 minutes or so.

The second batch won't gel as well as the first, but it's still full of nutrients that are tough to find elsewhere. Reducing it for a longer period of time will help it to gel. If you have the time try to get as many batches from these bones as possible. Remember, each batch will require more time reducing down to make it gel.

After everything is transferred into containers place them in the freezer. If you want to use one soon then set it in the fridge. The next day everything will have cooled leaving a layer of tallow or animal fat on the top. You can eat this or use it. It's full of healthy saturated fat that you can cook with. You can scoop it off with a spoon into another container. The remaining broth can be poured into ice cube trays to freeze into smaller easier to use cubes. If you want to prevent the fat from being in the broth you can strain your warm broth through cheese cloth prior to transferring to your final containers, but you will probably still get some in the final product.

To use the bone broth I make a simple soup. Take a few scoops of the gelatinized broth and put them into a pot. Add some water, a tablespoon of coconut oil for more healthy saturated fats, a few heaping dashes of ground turmeric and I dice up part of an onion. Bonus points if that onion is purple. A diced clove of garlic would also be great. Sometimes I add a little meat. Feel free to make what you want. I landed on this recipe because it is an easy way to include some healthy foods.

2.) Broccoli Sprouts – Make your own in the kitchen. Most people use wide mouth Mason jars and a straining lid from Amazon. I get my broccoli sprout seeds from Amazon. I scoop a tablespoon of seeds into a Mason jar, rinse the seeds with water and then let them soak for 12 hours. Everyday thereafter I rinse the seeds with clean water and drain. Set the jar with the lid down in a dish drying rack. This allows excess water to flow down. Set them in the Sun for a day or two and the leaves will change from pale green to dark green. After 4 or 5 days the sprouts should be ready to eat.

They will taste gross especially, the way I make them. Pour out the sprouts onto a plate, cover liberally with ground mustard, chop up and eat with a fork. The flavor is pretty strong. Remember, this provides nutrients such as glucoraphanin, sulforaphane and myrosinase in large amounts that you can't get anywhere else.

3.) Homemade Nut Butters – Tired of peanut butter and don't want to spend a fortune on store bought almond or cashew butter? All you need is a food processor with a fine grit blade and some of your favorite nuts. You'll need to experiment on percentages as different nuts contain different amounts of oil. Those with less oil don't turn into butter unless they are mixed with something else. Almonds have enough oil to mix with other nuts. My favorite mix is about 2 parts walnuts to 3 parts almonds with a dash of maple syrup. I love peanut butter, but have found that it has such a strong and unique flavor that it does not taste the best with other nuts. It does, however, taste delicious with a little chocolate and honey.

4.) Live far far away from airports – Since airplanes and jets still use leaded fuel this pollution contaminates neighborhoods near airports. In one unusual instance a plane in flight dumped jet fuel on a playground near the airport injuring over 60 people.[119] Most of the environmental impacts are not as obvious.

5.) Reduce Prescriptions – Wean yourself off of the need for prescriptions by gradually improving your health. This may be harder than it seems, but if your medications are for chronic self-induced health concerns you should be able to change your lifestyle so you can start to get healthier.

6.) My Top 6 Foods – Incorporate these foods into your diet as they contain diverse nutrients that other foods do not have or in such large amounts that are hard to find.

Eggs
Walnuts
Broccoli
Mushrooms
Garlic
Sweet Potato

POST SCRIPT

If you've made it this far there is one final connection I want to share with you. Did you notice how the trends changed? Generations from yesterday died from things they either did not understand (germs) or could not control (it's hard to wash your hands if you don't have clean water). The major killers from the 1800's were all environmental. The victims had little choice in contracting an infection and few treatment options which led to death. The opposite is true now. Today, we die from ailments that we understand and are able to control. As mentioned earlier, the CDC estimates 40% of deaths are *preventable*. Most people are dying from something that starts from within. This is reflected in the overall change in our lives from prior generations to now; eating more and moving less.

It's infectious diseases versus chronic degenerative disease.

Take a step back and ponder this for a moment; our eating is not out of necessity. It is out of *desire*. I want a pizza. I want a plate of spaghetti. I want two cookies for dessert. I want to eat, eat, eat all day long. I want. I want. I want. We eat too much because we want to. We also are not active because we are lazy which is also something we *desire*. I don't want to work. I don't want to sweat. I want to sit in my comfy chair. I want someone else to do that for me…to take care of me.

Once you realize that your ailments today have more to do with your heart than they do with your body you will realize the root cause to most of your illnesses. Your health is your responsibility; not your doctor's, not your parents', not your community's, not your insurance company's, not the president's or the FDA's or Department of Agriculture's. Your health is yours and it starts with the attitude of your heart. Are you going to worship your body by pleasing your senses?

If you answer yes then you know what to expect later in life.

If you answer no then I encourage you to worship something better than yourself.

FURTHER READING

The following books and websites are great sources of general information relating to the conditions and treatments mentioned. For specific data see the published journals referenced for the topic you're reviewing. The books I found most fascinating were Matthew Walker's Why We Sleep and Dumping Iron by P.D. Mangan. If you know someone with Alzheimer's Disease then you will want to read Max Lugavere's Genius Foods and The End of Alzheimer's by Dale Bredesen. All of the Nourishing books by Sally Fallon Morell's are excellent.

The Blue Zones book offers great insight, but misrepresents data and misses easy observations such as warm climate and sunshine that should be considered factors for living a long time. The data misrepresentation is for the purpose of leading people to a plant-based diet. How Not To Die by Michael Greger suffers from the same incorrect, unhealthy, over-emphasis of the false virtues of a plant-based diet. Needless to say, they contain unique nuggets of wisdom which warrants their inclusion on this list.

BOOKS

Blue Zones: 9 Lessons For Living Longer From the People Who've
        Lived the Longest by Dan Buettner
Brain Maker: The Power of Gut Microbes to Heal and Protect Your
        Brain for Life by David Perlmutter and Kristin Loberg
the Brain's Way of Healing: Remarkable Discoveries and Recoveries
        from the Frontiers of Neuroplasticity by Norman Doidge,
        M.D.
Breasts: A Natural and Unnatural History by Florence Williams
Deep Nutrition: Why Your Genes Need Traditional Food by
        Catherine Shanahan MD and Luke Shanahan
the Dental Diet: The Surprising Link Between Your Teeth, Real
        Food, and Life-Changing Natural Health by Dr. Steven Lin
Dumping Iron: How To Ditch This Secret Killer and Reclaim Your
        Health by P.D. Mangan
the End of Alzheimer's: The First Program to Prevent and Reverse
        Cognitive Decline by Dale Bredesen, M.D.

Genius Foods: Become Smarter, Happier, and More Productive
        While Protecting Your Brain for Life by Max Lugavere with
        Paul Grewal, M.D.
Grain Brain: The Surprising Truth About Wheat, Carbs and Sugar by
        Dr. David Perlmutter
How Not To Die by Michael Greger M.D.
Influenza: The Hundred-Year Hunt To Cure the Deadliest Disease
        In History by Dr. Jeremy Brown
the Longevity Paradox: How To Die Young At A Ripe Old Age by
        Steven R. Gundry, MD.
Nourishing Broth: An Old-Fashioned Remedy for the Modern World
        by Sally Fallon Morell and Kaayla T. Daniel PhD, CCN
Nourishing Diets: How PALEO, and ANCESTRAL PEOPLES
        Really ATE by Sally Fallon Morell
the Salt Fix: Why the Experts Got It All Wrong and How Eating
        More Might Save Your Life by Dr. James DiNicolantonio
Tomatoland: How Modern Industrial Agriculture Destroyed Our
        Most Alluring Fruit by Barry Estabrook 1st ed.
Wheat Belly: Lose the Wheat, Lose the Weight, and Find Your Path
        Back to Health by William Davis
Why We Sleep: Unlocking the Power of Sleep and Dreams by
        Matthew Walker Ph.D

WEBSITES
bioflexlaser.com – Low Intensity Laser Therapy pioneers.
brainhq.com – A place to train the brain to keep it functioning well.
clinicaltrials.gov – Search active research studies.
drmalcolmkendrick.org – All about cardiovascular disease.
examine.com - Summaries of published research relating to
        supplements.
foundmyfitness.com – Nutritionist Rhonda Patrick M.D.'s website.
listeningcentre.org – Listening therapy based on the Tomatis Method.
ndb.nal.usda.gov/ndb/search/list – USDA nutrient database.
normandoidge.com – Website for the author of The Brain's Way of
        Healing and also The Brain That Changes Itself. Website has
        up to date info on discoveries and stories about healing the
        brain.
nutritionfacts.org – Often misleading, but some good general info.

phenol-explorer.eu/ - Collection of published research on
polyphenols.

quackwatch.org – Compilation of misleading health fads, physicians
and organizations.

recalls.gov/food – List of US food recalls.

sciencedaily.com – Aggregate site for published studies. Provides
brief summaries. Excellent place to find sources. Also,
phys.org, eurekalert.com and MedicalXpress.com.

selfhacked.com – One man's massive compilation of many
treatments.

whfoods.com – A collection of foods and nutrients. Can sort by food
to see its nutrients or nutrients to see foods it's in.

westonaprice.org – The Weston A. Price Foundation's page about
nutrition.

wikipedia.com – The internet encyclopedia; not to be taken at face
value, but has lots of sources. This is a good starting point to
get ideas.

REFERENCES

HEART DISEASE and STROKE 777,402 annual deaths

[1] Glyphosate Excretion Is Associated With Steatohepatitis and Advanced Liver Fibrosis In Patients With Fatty Liver Disease. Clinical Gastroenterology and Hepatology. Paul J. Mills. 2019.

[2] https://drmalcolmkendrick.org/

[3] A high menaquinone intake reduces the incidence of coronary heart disease. Gast GC, de Roos NM, Sluijs I, et al. 2009 Sep; 19(7): 504-510 journal Nutrition, Metabolism and Cardiovascular Disease.

[4] Antihypertensive effects and endothelial progenitor cell activation by intake of chicken collagen hydrolysate in pre- and mild-hypertension. Saiga-Egusa A, Iwai K, Hayakawa T, Takahata Y, Morimatsu F. Bioscience Biotechnology and Biochemistry. 2009 Feb;73(2):422-4.
https://www.ncbi.nlm.nih.gov/pubmed/19202283

[5] Absorption and effectiveness of orally administered low molecular weight collagen hydrolysate in rats. Watanabe-Kamiyama M, Shimizu M, Kamiyama S, et al. Journal of Agricultural and Food Chemistry. 2010 Jan 27;58(2):835-41.
https://www.ncbi.nlm.nih.gov/pubmed/19957932

[6] Cardiovascular Drug Reviews. Silvia Bradamante, Livia Barenghi, and Alessandro Villa. 22(3) 169–188.

[7] Resveratrol Prevents Hyperglycemia-induced Endothelial dDsfunction Via Activation of Adenosine Monophosphate-activated Protein Kinase. Qiang Xua, Xinzhong Hao, et al. Biochemical and Biophysical Research Communications. 388(2) 389-394. 16 October 2009.
https://www.sciencedirect.com/science/article/pii/S0006291X09015733

[8] Cardioprotection By Resveratrol: A Human Clinical Trial In Patients With Stable Coronary Artery Disease. Magyar, K., Halmosi, R., et al. Clinical Hemorheology and Microcirculation, 50(3) 179-187, 2012.
https://content.iospress.com/articles/clinical-hemorheology-and-microcirculation/ch1424.

[9] Calcium Intake From Diet and Supplements and the Risk of Coronary Artery Calcification and its Progression Among Older Adults: 10-Year Follow-up of the Multi-Ethnic Study of Atherosclerosis (MESA). John J.B. Anderson, Bridget Kruska, Joseph A.C. Delanay. JAHA Journal of the American Heart Association.October 11, 2016.

[10] Calcium supplements and cardiovascular risk: 5 years on. Mark J. Bolland, Andrew Grey and Ian R. Reid. 2013 October 4(5): 199-210. Journal – Therapeutic Advances in Drug Safety.

[11] Dr. Tadeusz Malinski in International Journal of Nanomedicine. Jan 2018.

[12] Article from The Lancet; Low-level lead exposure and mortality in US adults: a population-based cohort study. Bruce P. Lanphear, MD, Stephen Rauch, MPH, Peggy Auinger, MS, et. al. Volume 3, Issue 4, PE177-E184, April 01, 2018.

[13] Tanjaniina Laukkanen et al, Sauna bathing is associated with reduced

cardiovascular mortality and improves risk prediction in men and women: a prospective cohort study, *BMC Medicine* (2018).

[14] Walnuts Decrease Risk of Cardiovascular Disease: A Summary of Efficacy and Biologic Mechanisms. Penny M. Kris-Etherton. The Journal of Nutrition, Volume 144, Issue 4, 1 April 2014, Pages 547S-554S. https://academic.oup.com/jn/article/144/4/547S/4571627

[15] The Evidence for Saturated Fat and for Sugar Related to Coronary Heart Disease. DiNicolantonio, J.J., Lucan S.C., O'Keefe, J.H.; Progressive Cardiovascular Disease. 2016. Mar-Apr; 58(5):464-472. https://www.ncbi.nlm.nih.gov/pubmed/26586275

[16] Effect of dietary calcium and milk consumption on risk of thromboembolic stroke in older middle-aged men. The Honolulu Heart Program. Abbot RD, Curb JD, Rodriguez BL. 1996 May 27(5) 813-818. STROKE AHA Journal.

[17] Association of Skipping Breakfast With Cardiovascular and All-Cause Mortality. Shuang Rong, Linda G. Snetselaar, et al. Journal of the American College of Cardiology. Volume 73, Issue 16, April 2019. http://www.onlinejacc.org/content/73/16/2025.

[18] Impact of Changes In Heart Rate With Age On All-cause Death and Cardiovascular Events In 50-year-old Men From the General Population. Xiao-jing Chen, Salim Bary Barywani, et al. Open Heart 2019;6:e000856. https://openheart.bmj.com/content/6/1/e000856.

CANCER 598,038 annual deaths

[19] Biological and therapeutic effects of ortho-silicic acid and some ortho-silicic acid-releasing compounds: New perspectives for therapy. Lela Munjas Jurkić, Ivica Cepanec, et al. Nutrition & Metabolism. Volume 10, Article number: 2 (2013). https://www.ncbi.nlm.nih.gov/pmc/articles/PMC3546016/.

[20] A great article which summarizes other research and provides new conclusions; Walnuts Have Potential for Cancer Prevention and Treatment in Mice. W. Elaine Hardman. The Journal of Nutrition. 2014 Apr; 144(4): 555S–560S. https://academic.oup.com/jn/article/144/4/555S/4571631.

[21] Dietary walnut altered gene expressions related to tumor growth, survival, and metastasis in breast Cancer patients: A pilot clinical trial. W. Elaine Hardmana, Donald A.Primerano, et al., Nutrition Research. Online only as of 30 March 2019. Accepted for publication. I will need to follow up to see when this is printed. https://www.sciencedirect.com/science/article/pii/S0271531718311904?via%3Dihub.

[22] Consumption of a dark roast coffee blend reduces DNA damage in humans: results from a 4-week randomised controlled study. Schipp, Tulinska J., et al. European Journal of Nutrition. 2018 Nov 17. https://www.ncbi.nlm.nih.gov/pubmed/30448878.

[23] Dark coffee consumption protects human blood cells from spontaneous DNA damage. Gudrun Pahlkea, Eva Attakpah, et al. Journal of Functional Foods.

Volume 55, April 2019, Pages 285-295.
https://www.sciencedirect.com/science/article/pii/S1756464619300702?via%3Di
hub.

[24] Pomiferin, histone deacetylase inhibitor isolated from the fruits of *Maclura pomifera*. Il Hong Son, Ill-Min Chung, et al. Bioorganic and Medicinal Chemistry Letters. 17(2007) 4,753-4755.
https://personal.evangel.edu/badgers/Web/Osage/Pomiferin%20histone%20deac
etylase%20inhibitor.pdf

[25] https://gis.cdc.gov/cancer/USCS/DataViz.html.

[26] (Lycopene and the Lung. Lenore Arab, Susan Steck-Scott and Aaron T. Fleishauer. Experimental Biology and Medicine. November 1, 2002. Volume: 227 issue: 10, page(s): 894-899.

[27] Medicine (Baltimore) 2017 Jun; 96(22): e7049 Daily Sedentary time and its association with risk for colorectal cancer in adults: A dose-response meta-analysis of prospective cohort studies. Peng Ma, MD., Yonggang Yao, MD., Weili Sun, MD., et al. Taken from
https://www.ncbi.nlm.nih.gov/pmc/articles/PMC5459729/

[28] Contemporary Hormonal Contraception and the Risk of Breast Cancer, Lina S Morch Ph. D., Charlotte W. Skovlund., M. Sc., Philip C. Hannaford, M.D., Lisa Iversen, Ph. D., Shona Fielding, Ph. D., and Ojvind Lidegaard, D.M. Sci. New England Journal of Medicine 2017; 377:2228-2239, December 7, 2017.

[29] Dietary walnut altered gene expressions related to tumor growth, survival, and metastasis in breast cancer patients: a pilot clinical trial. Hardman WE, Primerano DA, et al. Nutrition Research. 2019 Jun;66:82-94.
https://www.ncbi.nlm.nih.gov/pubmed/30979659

[30] Flavonoid Derivative of Cannabis Demonstrates Therapeutic Potential in Preclinical Models of Metastatic Pancreatic Cancer. Michele Moreau, Udoka Ibeh, et al. Frontiers In Oncology. 2019; 9: 660.
https://www.ncbi.nlm.nih.gov/pmc/articles/PMC6663976/

[31] The Fruits of Maclura pomifera Extracts Inhibits Glioma Stem-Like Cell Growth and Invasion. Dan Zhao, Chengyun Yao, et al. Neurochemical Research. October 2013, Volume 38, Issue 10, pp 2105–2113.
https://link.springer.com/article/10.1007/s11064-013-1119-8.

[32] Viral targeting of non-muscle invasive bladder cancer and priming of anti-tumour immunity following intravesical Coxsackievirus A21. Nicola E Annels, David Mansfield, et al. Clinical Cancer Research. July 4 2019 DOI: 10.1158/1078-0432.CCR-18-4022.
https://clincancerres.aacrjournals.org/content/early/2019/06/29/1078-
0432.CCR-18-4022#.

[33] A prospective study of tea drinking temperature and risk of esophageal squamous cell carcinoma. Farhad Islami, Hossein Poustchi, Akram Pourshams, et al. International Journal of Cancer Volume 0, Issue 0. (published online 20 March 2019. Not yet published in print.)
https://onlinelibrary.wiley.com/doi/full/10.1002/ijc.32220.

[34] Dietary Tomato Paste Protects against Ultraviolet Light–Induced Erythema in Humans. Wilhelm Stahl, Ulrike Heinrich, Sheila Wiseman, et al. The Journal of

Nutrition, Volume 131, Issue 5, May 2001, Pages 1449–1451. https://academic.oup.com/jn/article/131/5/1449/4686953.
[35] Safety and Efficacy of Oral Polypodium leucotomos Extract in Healthy Adult Subjects. Mark S. Nestor, MD, PhD., Brian Berman, MD, PhD. and Nicole Swenson, DO. Journal of Clinical and Aesthetic Dermatology. 2015 Feb; 8(2): 19–23. https://www.ncbi.nlm.nih.gov/pmc/articles/PMC4345929/.
[36] Polypodium Leucotomos - An Overview of Basic Investigative Findings. Brian Berman MD PhD., Charles Ellis MD. and Craig Elmets MD. Journal of Drugs and Dermatology. February 2016. 15(2): 224.
[37] Ohkuma N, Kajita S, Iizuka H. Superoxide dismutase in epidermis: its relation to keratinocyte proliferation. *Journal of Dermatology*. 1987;14(6):562–568.
[38] Galeotti T, Borrello S, Seccia A. Superoxide dismutase content in human epidermis and squamous cell epithelioma. *Archives of Dermatological Research*. 1980;267(1):83–86.
[39] http://lpi.oregonstate.edu/mic/health-disease/skin-health/vitamin-A see the Photoaging section.
[40] Improvement of naturally aged skin with vitamin a (retinaol). Kafi R, Kwak HS, Schumacher WE, Cho S, Hanft VN et al. Arch Dermatol 2007 May; 143(5):606-12.
[41] A Review of the Diagnosis and Treatment of Ochratoxin A Inhalational Exposure Associated with Human Illness and Kidney Disease including Focal Segmental Glomerulosclerosis. Janette H. Hope and Bradley E. Hope. Journal of Environmental and Public Health. Volume 2012, Article ID 835059, 10 pages. https://www.hindawi.com/journals/jeph/2012/835059/.
[42] *Hypothesis*: Does ochratoxin A cause testicular cancer? Gary G. Schwartz. Cancer Causes & Control. February 2002, Volume 13, Issue 1, pp 91–100. https://link.springer.com/article/10.1023%2FA%3A1013973715289.

ACCIDENTS 161,374 annual deaths

[43] https://www.cdc.gov/niosh/motorvehicle/resources/crashdata/facts.html
[44] https://www.cdc.gov/motorvehiclesafety/impaired_driving/states.html.
[45] Muscle Nerve; 2016 Apr; 53(4): 598-607. Magnetic stimulation supports muscle and nerve regeneration after trauma in mice; Meline N. L. Stolting, MD, PhD., Anne Sophie Arnold, PhD., Deana Haralampieva, M. Sc., et al. https://www.ncbi.nlm.nih.gov/pmc/articles/PMC5130145/
[46] https://iowadot.gov/crashanalysis/top200.aspx.

RESPIRATORY DISEASE 154,596 annual deaths

[47] https://icat.iowadot.gov/.
[48] https://www.nhtsa.gov/recalls
[49] Vitamin C Supplementation for Pregnant Smoking Women and Pulmonary Function in their Newborn Infants: A Randomized Clinical Trial; Cindy T.

McEvoy, Diane Schilling, Nakia Clay, et al, JAMA 2014 MAY; 311(20):2074-2082. https://www.ncbi.nlm.nih.gov/pubmed/24838476.
[50] Chen Y, Blaser MJ. Inverse Associations of Helicobacter pylori With Asthma and Allergy. Arch Intern Med. 2007;167(8):821–827. https://jamanetwork.com/journals/jamainternalmedicine/fullarticle/412291.
[51] Reduction of exercise-induced asthma oxidative stress by lycopene, a natural antioxidant. I. Neuman H., Nahum A., Ben-Amotz., Allergy Volume 55, Issue 12. https://onlinelibrary.wiley.com/doi/full/10.1034/j.1398-9995.2000.00748.x.
[52] https://www.citylab.com/environment/2019/04/mapping-where-traffic-air-pollution-hurts-children-most/587170/.
[53]https://airnow.gov/index.cfm?action=airnow.local_state&stateid=16&mapcenter=0&tabs=0.
[54] Association of Changes in Air Quality With Incident Asthma in Children in California, 1993-2014. Erika Garcia, PhD; Kiros T. Berhane, PhD; Talat Islam, PhD; et al. JAMA. 2019;321(19):1906-1915. https://jamanetwork.com/journals/jama/article-abstract/2733972.
[55] https://eurekalert.org/pub_releases/2019-06/wtsi-flm061419.php.
[56] Transient relief of asthma symptoms during jaundice: a possible beneficial role of bilirubin. Takashi Ohrui, Hiroyasu Yasuda, et al. Tohoku Journal of Experimental Medicine. 2003 Mar;199(3):193-6. https://www.jstage.jst.go.jp/article/tjem/199/3/199_3_193/_pdf/-char/en.
[57] The upper-airway microbiota and loss of asthma control among asthmatic children. Yanjiao Zhou, Avraham Beigelman, et al. Nature Communications. Volume 10, Article number: 5714 (2019). https://www.nature.com/articles/s41467-019-13698-x#citeas.

ALZHEIMERS, DEMENTIA & COGNITIVE DECLINE 116,103 annual deaths

[58] Aβ and tau prion-like activities decline with longevity in the Alzheimer's disease human brain. Atsushi Aoyagi, Carlo Condello, et al. Science Translational Medicine. 01 May 2019: Vol. 11, Issue 490. https://stm.sciencemag.org/content/11/490/eaat8462, and here is a synopsis of the study https://neurosciencenews.com/alzheimers-double-prion-disorder-13010.
[59] Dementia Mortality in the United States, 2000–2017 by Ellen A. Kramarow, Ph.D., and Betzaida Tejada-Vera, M.S. National Vital Statistics Report. Volume 68, Number 2 March 14, 2019. https://www.cdc.gov/nchs/data/nvsr/nvsr68/nvsr68_02-508.pdf
[60] Reciprocal modulation between amyloid precursor protein and synaptic membrane cholesterol revealed by live cell imaging. Claire E. DelBove, Claire E. Strothman, et al. Neurobiology of Disease. Volume 127, July 2019, Pages 449-461. https://www.sciencedirect.com/science/article/pii/S0969996118306934.
[61]https://www.sciencedaily.com/releases/2019/04/190423113951.htm.
[62] A prospective study of physical activity and cognitive decline in elderly women:

women who walk. Yaffe, K., Barnes, D., et al. Archives of Internal Medicine. 2001 Jul 23;161(14):1703-8. https://www.ncbi.nlm.nih.gov/pubmed/11485502.

[63] A longitudinal study of cardiorespiratory fitness and cognitive function in healthy older adults. Barnes, D., Yaffe, K., et al. Journal of the American Geriatrics Society. 2003 Apr;51(4):459-65. https://www.ncbi.nlm.nih.gov/pubmed/12657064.

[64] Physical activity, APOE genotype, and dementia risk: findings from the Cardiovascular Health Cognition Study., Podewils, LJ., Guallar, E., et al., American Journal of Epidemiology. 2005 Apr 1;161(7):639-51. https://www.ncbi.nlm.nih.gov/pubmed/15781953.

[65] Exercise is associated with reduced risk for incident dementia among persons 65 years of age and older. Larson EB., Wang L., et al. Annals of Internal Medicine. 2006 Jan 17;144(2):73-81.

[66] Exercise Influence on Hippocampal Function: Possible Involvement of Orexin-A. Chieffi, Sergio., Monda, Marcellino., et al. Frontiers in Physiology, 2017;8:85. https://www.frontiersin.org/articles/10.3389/fphys.2017.00085/full.

[67] Effects of DHA Supplementation on Hippocampal Volume and Cognitive Function in Older Adults with Mild Cognitive Impairment, Zhang, YP; Miao, R. Journal of Alzheimer's Disease, 2017;55(2):497-507. https://www.ncbi.nlm.nih.gov/pubmed/27716665.

[68] Taken from https://www.nature.com/articles/d41586-018-02391-6.

[69] Spirulina Promotes Stem Cell Genesis and Protects against LPS Induced Declines in Neural Stem Cell Proliferation. Adam Bachstetter, Jennifer Jernberg, Andrea Schlunk, et al. PLoS One: 2010; 5(5) e10496. https://www.researchgate.net/publication/44593502_Spirulina_Promotes_Stem_Cell_Genesis_and_Protects_against_LPS_Induced_Declines_in_Neural_Stem_Cell_Proliferation.

[70] Midlife cardiovascular fitness and dementia. A 44-year longitudinal population study in women. Helena Hörder, Ingmar Skoog, et al. Neurology. April 10, 2018; 90 (15). News article about the study https://www.usatoday.com/story/news/nation/2018/03/14/highly-fit-middle-age-women-nearly-90-less-likely-develop-dementia-decades-later-study-finds/425210002/.

[71] Sedentary behavior associated with reduced medial temporal lobe thickness in middle-aged and older adults. Prabha Siddarth, Alison C. Burggren, Harris A. Eyre. April 12, 2018. http://journals.plos.org/plosone/article?id=10.1371/journal.pone.0195549

[72] Synergistic neuroprotection by coffee components eicosanoyl-5-hydroxytryptamide and caffeine in models of Parkinson's disease and DLB. Ran Yan, Jie Zhang, Hye-Jin Park, et all; Proceedings of the National Academy of Sciences, Dec 3, 2018. Published online prior to print. https://www.pnas.org/content/early/2018/11/26/1813365115

[73] Scientific Reports. 2018 Feb 2;8(1):2246. Lundgaard, I., Wang, W., Eberhard, A., Nedergaard, M. Beneficial effects of low alcohol exposure, but adverse effects of high alcohol intake on glymphatic function. https://www.ncbi.nlm.nih.gov/pubmed/29396480.

[74] Explanation regarding the doses https://www.livescience.com/61659-does-alcohol-clean-brain.html

[75] Omega-3 polyunsaturated fatty acids promote amyloid-β clearance from the brain through mediating the function of the glymphatic system. Huixia Ren., Chuanming Luo., et al. The FASEB Journal. Published online October 1, 2016. https://www.fasebj.org/doi/full/10.1096/fj.201600896.

[76] Blood-brain barrier breakdown is an early biomarker of human cognitive dysfunction. Daniel A. Nation, Melanie D. Sweeney. et. al. Nature Medicine (2019). 14 January 2019. https://www.nature.com/articles/s41591-018-0297-y#Abs1

[77] Fibrinogen Induces Microglia-Mediated Spine Elimination and Cognitive Impairment in an Alzheimer's Disease Model. Mario Merlini, Victoria A. Rafalski, Pamela E. Rios Coronado, et. al. Neuron. 2019 Mar 20;101(6):1099-1108. https://www.ncbi.nlm.nih.gov/pubmed/30737131. A summary of the study can be found at https://www.sciencedaily.com/releases/2019/02/190205115419.htm

[78] Porphyromonas gingivalis in Alzheimer's disease brains: Evidence for disease causation and treatment with small-molecule inhibitors. Stephen S. Dominy, Casey Lynch, Florian Ermini, et. al. Science Advances. 23 January 2019; Vol. 5 no. 1; http://advances.sciencemag.org/content/5/1/eaau3333

[79] Herp Viruses and Senile Dementia: First Population Evidence for a Causal Link. Itzhaki, RF., Lathe, R. Journal of Alzheimer's Disease. 2018; 64(2):363-366. https://www.ncbi.nlm.nih.gov/pubmed/29889070

[80] The Viral protein Corona Directs Viral Pathogenesis and Amyloid Aggregation. Kariem Ezzat, Maria Pernemalm, et al. Nature Communications 10, Article number: 2331 (2019). https://www.nature.com/articles/s41467-019-10192-2.

[81] Role of Walnuts in Maintaining Brain Health with Age. Shibu M. Poulose, Marshall G. Miller, Barbara Shukitt-Hale. The Journal of Nutrition, Volume 144, Issue 4, 1 April 2014, Pages 561S–566S. https://academic.oup.com/jn/article/144/4/561S/4571638

[82] Exercise-linked FNDC5/irisin rescues synaptic plasticity and memory defects in Alzheimer's models. Nature Medicine. 25, 165 – 175. 2019. Michael V. Lourenco, Rudimar L. Frozza, Guilherme B. de Freitas, et. al. https://www.nature.com/articles/s41591-018-0275-4

[83] Omega-3 Fatty Acid Docosahexaenoic Acid Increases SorLA/LR11, a Sorting Protein with Reduced Expression in Sporadic Alzheimer's Disease (AD): Relevance to AD Prevention. Qiu-Lan Ma, Bruce Teter, Oliver J. Ubeda, et al. Journal of Neuroscience 26 December 2007, 27 (52) 14299-14307. http://www.jneurosci.org/content/27/52/14299

[84] Effects of Transcranial Alternating Current Stimulation on Cognitive Functions in Healthy Young and Older Adults. Daria Antonenko, Miriam Faxel, et al. Neural Plasticity. Volume 2016, Article ID 4274127, 13 pages. https://www.hindawi.com/journals/np/2016/4274127/.

[85] Boosting Slow Oscillations During Sleep Potentiates Memory. Lisa Marshall, Halla Helgadóttir, et al. Nature. 444, 610–613. 2006. https://www.nature.com/articles/nature05278.

[86] Slow wave sleep disruption increases cerebrospinal fluid amyloid-β levels. Yo-El S Ju, Sharon J Ooms, et al. Brain. 2017 Aug; 140(8): 2104–2111.

https://academic.oup.com/brain/article/140/8/2104/3933862?searchresult=1.
[87] Anticholinergic Drug Exposure and the Risk of Dementia: A Nested Case-Control Study. Coupland CAC, Hill T, Dening T, et al. JAMA Intern Med. Published online June 24, 2019179(8):1084–1093. https://jamanetwork.com/journals/jamainternalmedicine/fullarticle/2736353.

DIABETES 80,058 annual deaths

[88] Reversal of type 2 diabetes: normalization of beta cell function in association with decreased pancreas and liver triacylglycerol. E.L. Lim, K.G. Hollingsworth, B.S. Aribisala, et. al. Diabetologia. 54(10) 2506-2514. October 2011. https://link.springer.com/article/10.1007%2Fs00125-011-2204-7
[89] High rates of diabetes reversal in newly diagnosed Asian Indian young adults with type 2 diabetes mellitus with intensive lifestyle therapy. Vijaya Sarathia, Anish Kolly, H.B. Chaithanya, et. al., Journal of Natural Science, Biology and Medicine. 8(1) 60-63. 2017. http://www.jnsbm.org/article.asp?issn=0976-9668;year=2017;volume=8;issue=1;spage=60;epage=63;aulast=Sarathi
[90] Pterostilbene Impact On Retinal Endothelial Cells Under High Glucose Environment. Hongjie Shen and Hua Rong. International Journal of Clinical Experimental Pathology. 2015; 8(10): 12589–12594. https://www.ncbi.nlm.nih.gov/pmc/articles/PMC4680394/.
[91] Impaired Insulin Signaling in Human Adipocytes After Experimental Sleep Restriction: A Randomized, Crossover Study. Josiane L. Broussard, PhD; David A. Ehrmann, MD., et al. Ann Intern Med. 2012;157(8):549-557. https://annals.org/aim/article-abstract/1379773/impaired-insulin-signaling-human-adipocytes-after-experimental-sleep-restriction-randomized?searchresult=1
[92] A1 beta-casein milk protein and other environmental pre-disposing factors for type 1 diabetes. J. S. J. Chia, J. L. McRae., et al. Nutrition and Diabetes. 2017 May; 7(5): e274. https://www.ncbi.nlm.nih.gov/pmc/articles/PMC5518798/.

INFLUENZA & PNEUMONIA 12,000 – 79,000 annual deaths

[93] https://www.cdc.gov/flu/about/burden/2017-2018.htm.
[94] Data from https://www.cdc.gov/flu/about/burden/past-seasons.html.
[95] High Ferritin, but Not Hepcidin, Is Associated with a Poor Immune Response to an Influenza Vaccine in Hemodialysis Patients. Eiselt J.a., Kielberger L.a., Sedláčková T., et al. Nephron Clinical Practice. 2010;115:c147–c153. https://www.karger.com/Article/Abstract/312878.
[96] https://msutoday.msu.edu/news/2019/food-additive-may-influence-how-well-flu-vaccines-work/. The study was done using the flu, but the effects are likely to be applicable to many other types of infections
[97] https://sydney.edu.au/news-opinion/news/2019/04/24/eating-elderberries-could-help-minimise-influenza-symptoms.html. The University of Sydney

announced this through a press release. I have not been able to locate a published study related to this announcement.

[98] Elderberry flavonoids bind to and prevent H1N1 infection in vitro. Bill Roschek Jr., Ryan C. Fink, et al., Phytochemistry. Volume 70, Issue 10, July 2009, Pages 1255-1261. https://www.sciencedirect.com/science/article/abs/pii/S0031942209002386?via%3Dihub.

[99] Elderberry Supplementation Reduces Cold Duration and Symptoms in Air-Travellers: A Randomized, Double-Blind Placebo-Controlled Clinical Trial. Evelin Tiralongo, Shirley S. Wee, and Rodney A. Lea. Nutrients 2016, 8(4), 182. https://www.mdpi.com/2072-6643/8/4/182/htm.

[100] Clinical trial NCT03410862. https://clinicaltrials.gov/ct2/show/NCT03410862?term=nct03410862&rank=1.

KIDNEY DISEASE annual deaths 50,546

[101] Increased water intake reduces long-term renal and cardiovascular disease progression in experimental polycystic kidney disease. Sagar, P., Zhang, J., et al. PLoS One. 2019 Jan 2;14(1). https://journals.plos.org/plosone/article?id=10.1371/journal.pone.0209186.

[102] Kidney-targeted inhibition of protein kinase C-α ameliorates nephrotoxic nephritis with restoration of mitochondrial dysfunction. Nino Kvirkvelia, Michael P. Madaio, et al. Kidney International. August 2018Volume 94, Issue 2, Pages 280-291. https://www.kidney-international.org/article/S0085-2538(18)30181-9/fulltext.

TRENDS

[103] Ageing and the gut. A.L. D'Souza. Postgraduate Medical Journal. 2007 Jan; 83(975): 44–53. https://www.ncbi.nlm.nih.gov/pmc/articles/PMC2599964/

[104] Do Centenarians Die Healthy? An Autopsy Study. Andrea M. Berzlanovich, Wolfgang Keil, Thomas Waldhoer, et. al., The Journals of Gerontology: Series A, Volume 60, Issue 7, 1 July 2005, Pages 862–865. https://academic.oup.com/biomedgerontology/article/60/7/862/539576

[105] Season of Birth and Exceptional Longevity: Comparative Study of American Centenarians, Their Siblings, and Spouses. Leonid A. Gavrilov and Natalia S. Gavrilova. Journal of Aging Research, Volume 2011, article ID 104616. https://www.hindawi.com/journals/jar/2011/104616/

[106] Composition and Comparison of the Ocular Surface Microbiome in Infants and Older Children. Kara M. Cavuoto, Santanu Banerjee, et al. Translational Vision Science and Technology. 2018 Nov; 7(6): 16. https://www.ncbi.nlm.nih.gov/pmc/articles/PMC6269136/

[107] https://ethics.harvard.edu/blog/new-prescription-drugs-major-health-risk-few-

offsetting-advantages

[108] The fixed combination of valerian and hops (Ze91019) acts via a central adenosine mechanism. Schellenberg, R., Sauer, S., Abourashed, E.A., et. al. Planta Medica 2004 Jul;70(7):594-597. https://www.ncbi.nlm.nih.gov/pubmed/15254851

[109] Effects of transcutaneous vagus nerve stimulation in individuals aged 55 years or above: potential benefits of daily stimulation. Beatrice Bretherton, Lucy Atkinson, et al. Aging (Albany NY). 2019; 11:4836-4857. https://doi.org/10.18632/aging.102074.

[110] Evaluation in vitro of AGE-crosslinks breaking ability of rosmarinic acid. Daniel Jean, Maryse Pouligon, Claude Dalle, Glycative Stress Research. 2015; 2 (4): 204-207. http://www.toukastress.jp/webj/article/2015/GS15-26.pdf

[111] Serum ferritin is an important inflammatory disease marker, as it is mainly a leakage product from damaged cells. Douglas B. Kell and Etheresia Pretorius. Metallomics. Issue 4, 2014. https://pubs.rsc.org/en/content/articlelanding/2014/mt/c3mt00347g#!divAbstract.

[112] The Aging of Iron Man. Azhaar Ashraf, Maryam Clark, and Po-Wah So. Frontiers In Aging Neuroscience., 12 March 2018. https://www.frontiersin.org/articles/10.3389/fnagi.2018.00065/full.

[113] Old age-associated phenotypic screening for Alzheimer's disease drug candidates identifies sterubin as a potent neuroprotective compound from Yerba santa. Wolfgang Fischer, Antonio Currais, Zhibin Liang, et al. Redox Biology. Volume 21, February 2019. https://www.sciencedirect.com/science/article/pii/S2213231718311996?via%3Dihub

[114] The role of zinc in selective neuronal death after transient global cerebral ischemia. Koh JY1, Suh SW, et al. Science. 1996 May 17;272(5264):1013-6. https://www.ncbi.nlm.nih.gov/pubmed/8638123.

[115] The Essential Toxin: Impact of Zinc on Human Health. Laura M. Plum, Lothar Rink and Hajo Haase. International Journal of Environmental Research and Public Health 2010, 7(4), 1342-1365. https://www.ncbi.nlm.nih.gov/pmc/articles/PMC2872358/

[116] Taken from https://www.sciencealert.com/remote-tribes-living-in-the-amazon-are-healthier-than-you-as-they-age which was taken from https://jamanetwork.com/journals/jamacardiology/article-abstract/2713959

[117] Timing of blood pressure measurement related to caffeine consumption. Mort, JR., Kruse, HR., Annal Pharmacotherapy; 2008 Jan; 42(1)105-110. Dec 19. https://www.ncbi.nlm.nih.gov/pubmed/18094346.

[118] Press release with study to be presented later, not sure if it will be published. https://www.acc.org/about-acc/press-releases/2019/03/07/08/56/a-nap-a-day-keeps-high-blood-pressure-at-bay

[119] https://www.nbcnews.com/news/us-news/17-kids-injured-after-delta-jet-dumps-fuel-l-playground-n1115586

9 781794 825659